Skin Lesions

A practical guide to diagnosis, management and minor surgery

Julia Schofield
MRCP (UK) MRCGP
Consultant Dermatologist, St Albans and Hemel Hempstead
NHS Hospitals Trust, Herts

and

Roger Kneebone
FRCS FRCSEd MRCGP
General Practitioner, Trowbridge, Wilts

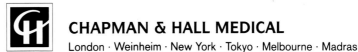

CHAPMAN & HALL MEDICAL
London · Weinheim · New York · Tokyo · Melbourne · Madras

Published by Chapman & Hall, 2–6 Boundary Row, London SE1 8HN, UK

Chapman & Hall, 2–6 Boundary Row, London SE1 8HN, UK

Blackie Academic & Professional, Wester Cleddens Road, Bishopbriggs, Glasgow G64 2NZ, UK

Chapman & Hall GmbH, Pappelallee 3, 69469 Weinheim, Germany

Chapman & Hall USA, 115 Fifth Avenue, New York, NY 10003, USA

Chapman & Hall Japan, ITP-Japan, Kyowa Building, 3F, 2-2-1 Hirakawacho, Chiyoda-ku, Tokyo 102, Japan

Chapman & Hall Australia, 102 Dodds Street, South Melbourne, Victoria 3205, Australia

Chapman & Hall India, R. Seshadri, 32 Second Main Road, CIT East, Madras 600 035, India

First edition 1996

© 1996 Julia Schofield and Roger Kneebone

Designed and formatted by Geoffrey and Marion Wadsley
Typeset in 10/12pt Palatino
Printed in Hong Kong by Dua Hua Printing Press Co., Ltd.

ISBN 0 412 63140 7

A catalogue record for this book is available from the British Library

Library of Congress Catalog Card Number: 95-71851

Contents

Foreword

For many doctors, 'skins' is the unkindest speciality of all. As undergraduates we may have formed the impression that the skin was a fickle and irrational organ, subject to unpronounceable diseases each a master of disguise, to be tamed only by those with a photographic memory, a fondness for Latin and Greek, and a magician's repertoire of spells, potions and incantations. Patients on the other hand, however impressed they might be by our knowledge of how their insides work, usually expect the management of lesions and rashes in full view on the surface of their bodies to be a simple affair. Those who find themselves 'doctors of first contact' – GP Principals and Registrars, Casualty Officers and junior hospital doctors – will welcome this *vade-mecum* which demystifies everyday dermatology and takes most of the worry out of dealing with lumps and bumps.

Confronted with a skin lesion (and the patient who sports it), the doctor finds a string of questions pressing for answers. What is it? Does it matter? Could it, or should it, be left alone? Or referred? Shall I remove it? Even if I'm not sure what it is? What would be the best technique? Suppose when the histology comes back I find I've incompletely excised a malignant melanoma...

Against this paralysing litany of self-doubt Julia Schofield and Roger Kneebone provide the antidote of common sense. Their book is as reassuring as having a friendly consultant on hand in the minor ops theatre to advise. It is systematic and comprehensive, yet eminently readable, practical and down to earth.

When I read a book intended to improve my knowledge and skills, I want it to be written, designed, presented and structured so as to fit comfortably with the ways I as an adult learn. I like to start with a bird's-eye view and a recapitulation of first principles on which subsequent learning can be based. I need the main ideas emphasized and reinforced at regular intervals. I hope there will be plenty of cross-referencing so that I can see important points from different perspectives. I feel reassured if the authors seem to have overcome the same problems I myself encounter. I like the writing to move seamlessly between the general and the particular, between principle and practice. And especially in a manual of dermatology dealing with visual material and manipulative skills, I want the text to be bolstered by good illustrations and effective graphic design, so that it becomes a pleasure to turn the pages.

The present authors bring a happy conjunction of writing ability and clinical experience to a book that more than satisfies these expectations.

As a member of their target audience, I consider that Julia Schofield and Roger Kneebone have done a great service to patients by ensuring that the doctors who treat their skin lesions have a competent grounding in diagnosis, management and risk assessment. From now on, I shall be far less anxious when a patient asks, 'Couldn't you just remove it for me, Doctor?'

Roger Neighbour, MA, FRCGP
General Practitioner
Abbots Langley, Hertfordshire

Preface

This book is written by a dermatologist who trained as a GP and a GP who has been a surgeon. We know from experience how difficult it can be to find quickly relevant guidance about skin lesions in an orthodox textbook, especially if you do not know what the lesion is. We have therefore adopted a different approach.

This is a practical handbook about dealing with clinical problems. Although it provides a large amount of factual information, the emphasis is on managing patients. It is not so much an academic treatise as a workshop manual, written from our own experience and reflecting our personal views.

As well as providing sections on basic dermatological knowledge and descriptions of specific techniques, the book tackles the following areas:

- how to manage a patient when you do not know the diagnosis;
- how to identify a lesion when you have seen it before but cannot remember its name;
- how to interpret the histology report.

The aim of the book is to help doctors make sensible management decisions about their patients, to deal with lesions themselves wherever possible and to refer to specialist colleagues when they are in doubt about what to do or how to do it. Strong links between GPs and their dermatological colleagues are the key to safe and rewarding management in this important area.

Acknowledgements

We wish to thank Len Cremore and Simon Tutty, our medical photographers, for the photographs which are an essential part of our book.

Special thanks are due to Paul Richardson, medical artist, who illustrated the sections on practical techniques. His attention to detail and cheerful willingness to make endless revisions have made working with him a particular pleasure.

We are grateful to Dr Frances Tatnall and Dr Paul Maurice for allowing us to use their clinical photographs.

We wish to acknowledge the kind permission of the following for allowing us to reproduce illustrations:

- The European Resuscitation Council (flow chart on resuscitation, Copyright European Resuscitation Council; Resuscitation 1994);
- Warecrest Ltd (rechargeable electrocautery machine);
- Seward Medical Ltd (surgical instruments);
- Limbs & Things Ltd, Bristol (simulated tissue);
- CryoTech Ltd (cryospray machine).

We are very grateful to Dr Roger Neighbour for his helpful criticism early on, and for writing the foreword to the book. We thank Dr Julia Newton-Bishop for her comments on the factual dermatological content and Dr Peter Adlard for his help with the final manuscript. But above all we owe an enormous debt of gratitude to Dr Peter Harney for his help with the style and presentation of our book. His encouragement, his gift for pruning and sharpening prose, his attention to detail and above all his generosity with his time have all been invaluable.

Finally, our thanks to all our dear families, who have given us such support while we have been away from them, writing this book.

Julia Schofield and Roger Kneebone
St Albans and Trowbridge, August 1995

Introduction

This is an unorthodox book, laid out in an unorthodox way. Many books on minor surgery concentrate on surgical techniques and how to learn them. In this book we have tried to give a wider view of the subject, based on our belief that diagnosis and management are as important as technical ability.

The book is written directly from the experience of two practising clinicians. It is a practical handbook written for busy doctors who need to identify a lesion quickly and decide how to manage it. There will always be different ways to approach any clinical problem and a book of this kind must inevitably seem didactic. Since too many alternatives can be confusing we have made definite recommendations in every case.

CLINICAL PRINCIPLES

*Golden rule: before removing a lesion you **must** try to make a diagnosis.*

Without a diagnosis you have no rational basis for deciding the best treatment. It is a dangerous practice to remove a lesion out of curiosity without first committing yourself to a provisional diagnosis.

*Golden rule: if you remove any tissue from a patient you **must** send it for histological examination.*

Only by doing this will you find out if your clinical diagnosis was correct. If it should prove to be wrong

you will need guidance on further management. This is provided in Chapter 3.

Golden rule: if in doubt, refer.

Work within your limitations and only carry out procedures about which you feel confident. Never be too proud to refer a patient to someone else. Sometimes you may be sure that a lesion is harmless and you will be able to reassure your patient that no treatment is required. At other times you may think a lesion needs to be removed but do not feel happy to do this yourself – the lesion may be unsuitable, it may be in a difficult site or you may simply not have confidence in your skills or your facilities. It is therefore essential to develop close links with local specialists.

The book is divided into two parts, the first dealing with relevant factual knowledge and the second with facilities and skills.

PART ONE: KNOWLEDGE

Basic dermatology

This concise account of the lesions you are likely to encounter starts with a guide to the prevalence of each lesion. Common things occur commonly. If you see a lesion you cannot identify it is much more likely to be an unfamiliar variant of a common condition than a rarity.

Because this is a practical book it is not exhaustive. We have left out most conditions that you would expect to see only once in a lifetime. The lesions are divided into benign and malignant. Each section is arranged with the commonest conditions first. Entries include a photograph of a typical lesion, some with a simple line drawing showing the part of the skin from which it arises. There follows a brief account of the lesion, with up-to-date information about management.

Guidance on management

This section provides a plan for the management of patients who present with a skin lesion, for although you should not **remove** a lesion without having made a diagnosis, you cannot refer every patient whose lesion you cannot identify. Managing uncertainty is an essential part of general practice. This section gives practical guidelines about dealing with uncertainty and using time as a diagnostic tool. It also highlights important conditions that are commonly confused.

The section ends with interpreting the histology report and what to do with the unexpected, e.g. an incompletely excised lesion, an unsuspected malignancy or something completely baffling. Guidance based on numerous real scenarios is given.

'Gallery' (pictorial quick reference guide)

Often you recognize a lesion but you cannot quite remember its name. A picture, however, may provide an instant diagnosis. The 'Gallery' is an atlas of conditions arranged in the same order as the clinical section. These pages are colour-coded for easy identification. Each 'Gallery' entry is laid out in the same way: name, photograph, a brief description and management. We have summarized possible treatments for each condition but have ended with our own recommendation in each case.

PART TWO: FACILITIES AND SKILLS

Background information

This section provides factual information and advice. It is intended as background reading and as a source of reference.
- Facilities
- Record keeping
- Audit
- Infection control
- Medicolegal considerations.

Practical skills

This section covers the essential skills you need to carry out the procedures referred to in the first part of the book. We have assumed very little previous knowledge. You may use this section to learn new skills or to refresh your memory about ones you have forgotten. Because these are practical techniques they require practical training to master them.
- **Anatomical hazards and pitfalls** points out important structures that may be at risk during minor surgical procedures.
- **Local anaesthesia** describes techniques used in minor skin surgery. It includes information about anaesthetic agents and gives guidance on what to do if things go wrong.
- **Basic surgical technique** covers the fundamental skills required to excise a lesion: planning the procedure, using instruments and needles, tying knots and suturing.
- **Dermatological techniques** describes curettage, cryotherapy, electrocautery and other practical skills.
- **Skills training** describes the use of simulated tissue for learning practical skills.

Part One

Knowledge

Chapter 1
Basic dermatology

INTRODUCTION

This chapter provides basic information about the clinical features and natural history of skin lesions. The chapter is in two sections: the first half describes benign conditions, the second half premalignant and malignant conditions. Particular attention is paid to the commoner lesions, although some of the more unusual ones are included for completeness.

A confident clinical diagnosis and a knowledge of the natural history of skin lesions are both vital when deciding whether surgical management of a particular lesion is appropriate. Where there is uncertainty about diagnosis it is better to avoid surgery. A patient with a poor cosmetic outcome is likely to be very dissatisfied if it becomes clear that the procedure was unnecessary, or inappropriate, or both.

CLASSIFICATION OF SKIN LESIONS

When examining a skin lesion and trying to make a diagnosis, it is helpful to think of the part of the skin from which the lesion is derived. This is illustrated in Figure 1.1.

Lesions can arise from various parts of the skin as follows:

- From **melanocytes** (Figure 1.2), e.g. freckle, lentigo, junctional melanocytic naevus, compound melanocytic naevus, intradermal melanocytic naevus, halo naevus, atypical melanocytic naevus, malignant melanoma. Melanocytes result in pigmentation, so many of these lesions, but not all, will be pigmented.

- From the **epidermis** (Figure 1.3), e.g. basal cell papilloma (also known as seborrhoeic wart or seborrhoeic keratosis), solar keratosis, Bowen's disease, squamous cell carcinoma. These arise from the upper part of the skin and so have a very superficial appearance.
- From **hair follicles** (Figure 1.4), e.g. epidermoid cysts (also known as pilar cysts). These are often incorrectly described as sebaceous cysts.
- From **fibroblasts** in the dermis (Figure 1.5), e.g. dermatofibroma (sometimes known as histiocytoma).
- From **blood vessels** in the dermis, e.g. spider naevi, Campbell de Morgan spots, pyogenic granuloma.

WHAT IS COMMON?

Table 1.1 shows the skin lesions most commonly removed in general practice. These data were obtained using histopathology reports of all lesions excised by general practitioners in south west Hertfordshire in a year.

BENIGN SKIN LESIONS

Pigmented melanocytic lesions

Melanocytes are present in the basal layer of the epidermis (Figure 1.1). The melanosomes in melanocytes produce the pigment melanin, responsible for skin pigmentation. The melanocytes of

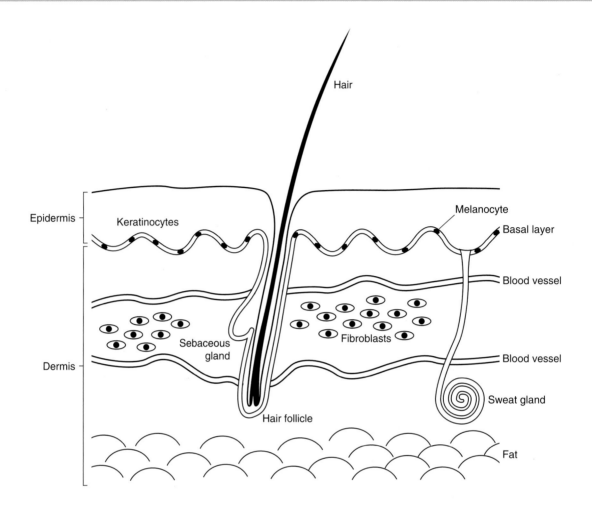

Figure 1.1 Diagrammatic representation of normal skin illustrating the various parts of the skin from which lesions are derived.

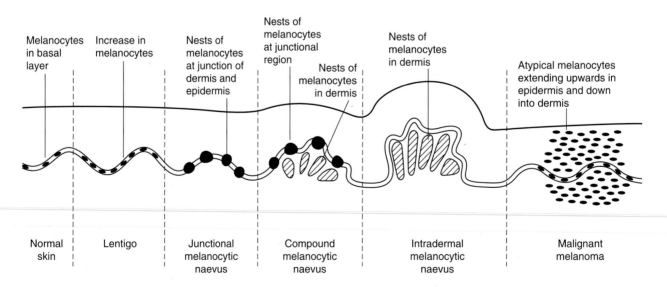

Figure 1.2 Diagrammatic representation of lesions derived from melanocytes.

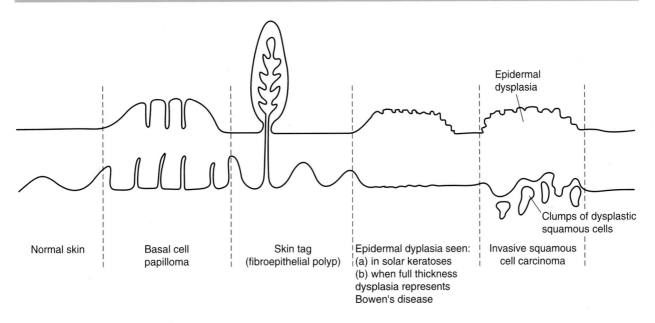

Epidermal
dysplasia

Clumps of dysplastic
squamous cells

Normal skin | Basal cell
papilloma | Skin tag
(fibroepithelial polyp) | Epidermal dyplasia seen:
(a) in solar keratoses
(b) when full thickness
dysplasia represents
Bowen's disease | Invasive squamous
cell carcinoma

Figure 1.3 Diagrammatic representation of lesions derived from the epidermis.

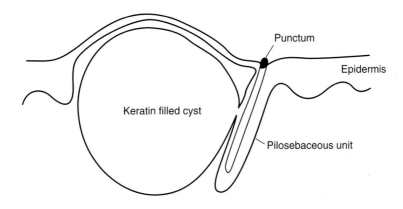

Punctum

Epidermis

Keratin filled cyst

Pilosebaceous unit

Figure 1.4 Diagrammatic representation of an epidermoid (pilar) cyst.

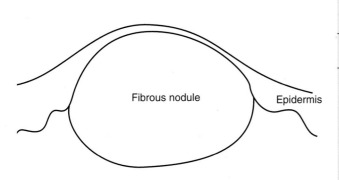

Fibrous nodule   Epidermis

Figure 1.5 Diagrammatic representation of a dermatofibroma, which is derived from fibroblasts of the dermis.

Table 1.1 Skin lesions most commonly removed in general practice	
Lesion	*Frequency (%)*
Melanocytic naevus	29
Basal cell papilloma (seborrhoeic keratosis)	24
Epidermoid cyst	16
Fibro-epithelial polyp (skin tags)	12
Dermatofibroma	5
Malignant lesions	2
Other, e.g. pyogenic granuloma	12

dark-skinned people produce more melanin than the melanocytes of fair-skinned people.

FRECKLES (EPHELIDES)

Freckles are pigmented macules that are usually 1–3 mm in diameter (Figure 1.6).

Typically they start to appear in childhood. They do not occur as a result of an increase in melanocytes. Rather, the melanosomes in the melanocytes of the freckle produce melanin much more readily in response to sunlight than the melanosomes in the surrounding skin.

Management

Most people with freckles have them in large numbers. While some consider them a cosmetic nuisance, treatment is inappropriate.

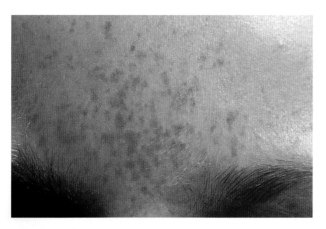

Figure 1.6 Freckles.

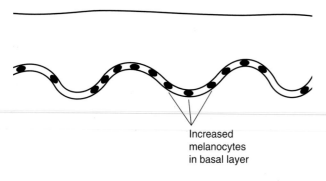

Figure 1.7 Diagrammatic representation of a lentigo.

Increased melanocytes in basal layer

Don't forget

Axillary freckling and café-au-lait patches are markers of neurofibromatosis.

LENTIGO

This is also a small pigmented macule (1–3 mm) but here the increase in pigmentation is due to an increase in the number of melanocytes in the basal layer (Figure 1.7).

Unlike freckles, these may be solitary, and do not darken as much after sun exposure (Figure 1.8).

It may be very difficult to distinguish a lentigo from a junctional naevus (p. 7). Multiple lentigines occur in the elderly on sun-exposed skin. These are called solar lentigines (Figures 1.9, 1.10).

Management

These lesions are usually very small and best left alone. Excision of a small lentigo leaves a scar much bigger than the original lesion. Larger lesions (5–10 mm diameter) occurring on the sun-damaged skin of the elderly may look worrying. In this group you may wish to arrange referral for a dermatological opinion for diagnostic confirmation. In the case of a lentigo on the face (Figure 1.11) it is important to consider the possible diagnosis of Hutchinson's freckle, which is also known as lentigo maligna. This premalignant melanocytic lesion is discussed in more detail later (p. 22).

Don't forget

Multiple lentigines presenting in childhood can be a cutaneous marker of systemic abnormalities, e.g. Peutz–Jeghers syndrome.

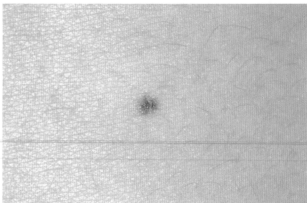

Figure 1.8 Lentigo.

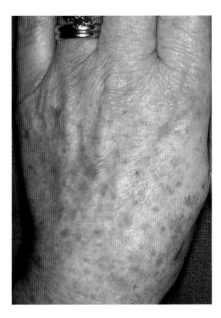

Figure 1.9 Multiple solar lentigines on the back of the hand.

Figure 1.10 Multiple solar lentigines on the back.

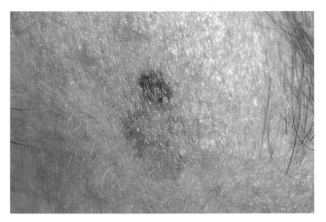

Figure 1.11 Lentigo on the face which could be an early Hutchinson's freckle (lentigo maligna).

Benign melanocytic naevi

The term 'mole', if used, should be reserved for this group of lesions. The term melanoma is best avoided when describing benign melanocytic naevi as it may cause confusion with malignant melanoma. Basal cell papillomas and solar keratoses are better referred to as keratoses rather than moles.

Benign melanocytic naevi are common, usually appearing in childhood and puberty. In later life these naevi disappear and it is rare to see melanocytic lesions in the elderly. Basal cell papillomas (p. 12) are much more frequent in this age group.

It is quite common to find 30–40 naevi, usually occurring on light-exposed skin. The fair-skinned, those with a family history of moles, and those with a history of increased sun exposure in childhood are more likely to have large numbers.

A melanocytic naevus usually evolves through three stages: from a new junctional naevus to a compound naevus and finally to a mature intradermal naevus. The clinical features of these three lesions are different. Complete evolution through the stages does not always occur and some people have many melanocytic naevi of different types. Sometimes a melanocytic naevus will develop a halo of depigmentation and then disappear (halo naevus, p. 9).

JUNCTIONAL MELANOCYTIC NAEVUS

This is due to melanocytic proliferation at the junction of the dermis and epidermis, hence the term 'junctional' (Figure 1.12).

Clinical features

A junctional naevus is typically flat and brown (Figure 1.13). It may be irregularly pigmented. It is sometimes difficult to tell a new junctional naevus from a malignant melanoma.

7

Management

If you are confident of the diagnosis there is no need to excise junctional naevi. If the patient is keen to have the lesion removed, this is best done by ellipse excision with a 2 mm margin (p. 111). If there is the slightest possibility of malignant melanoma you should refer the patient urgently for a dermatological opinion.

Don't forget

Be careful about making a diagnosis of a junctional naevus if the lesion has appeared for the first time in a patient over the age of 40, is growing rapidly, has an irregular border or is variably pigmented. With any of these features the diagnosis could be malignant melanoma.

COMPOUND MELANOCYTIC NAEVUS

In this lesion many of the proliferating naevus cells (nests) have dropped into the dermis. This pushes up the overlying epidermis, resulting in a raised lesion (Figure 1.14). Since melanocytic proliferation at the dermo-epidermal junction continues, the lesion remains pigmented.

Clinical features

This type of naevus is raised and usually pigmented (Figure 1.15).

Because it is easily caught or knocked, causing bleeding, excision is often requested.

Management

Shave excision with or without cautery avoids suturing and usually gives a good cosmetic result (p. 119). However, patients should be warned that pigmentation of the scar is not uncommon, that occasionally the naevus recurs and that if there were any hairs in the lesion these may regrow at the site of the scar.

Ellipse excision inevitably leaves a linear scar and should be avoided if possible. Before proceeding with ellipse excision be sure that the cosmetic result will be acceptable to the patient.

Again, if there is the slightest concern about malignant melanoma you should refer the patient to a dermatologist.

Don't forget

Shave excision biopsy is the wrong procedure if the lesion is subsequently shown to be a malignant melanoma. Similarly a large diagnostic ellipse excision is unacceptable if a shave excision would have sufficed.

INTRADERMAL MELANOCYTIC NAEVUS

In this lesion the junctional activity is no longer present and the naevus is predominantly in the dermis. These lesions are therefore raised. Because of the lack of junctional activity there is often no pigment (Figure 1.16).

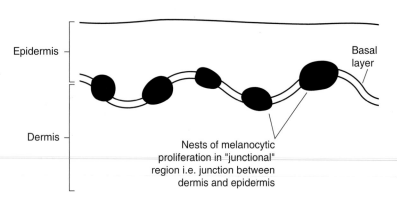

Figure 1.12 Diagrammatic representation of a junctional melanocytic naevus.

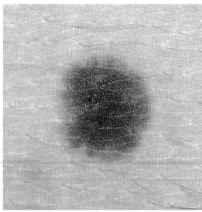

Figure 1.13 Junctional melanocytic naevus.

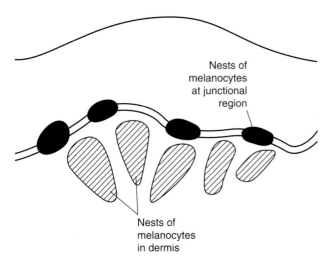

Figure 1.14 Diagrammatic representation of a compound melanocytic naevus.

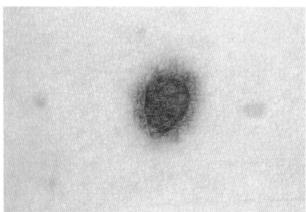

Figure 1.15 Compound melanocytic naevus.

Clinical features

These are common, particularly on the face of young and middle-aged women. Raised and typically non-pigmented, they may have hairs growing out of them (Figure 1.17). They are stable and unchanging but are often considered a cosmetic nuisance.

Management

Intradermal naevi lend themselves well to shave excision (p. 119). In particular, because of the lack of pigment, repigmentation of the scar is not a problem. However you should warn your patient that the lesion may recur and that the hairs may regrow.

Clinical confusion

Sometimes the pale, rather cystic appearance on the face may suggest a basal cell carcinoma. However an intradermal naevus will usually have been present unchanged for a long time, making the diagnosis of basal cell carcinoma unlikely. Since shave excision is the wrong treatment for a basal cell carcinoma, you should refer if the diagnosis is in doubt.

HALO NAEVUS (SUTTON'S NAEVUS)

Halo naevi usually occur in young adults and are often a source of considerable anxiety to patients and doctor alike. Here there is a localized immunological response to the pigment cells in and around the melanocytic naevus.

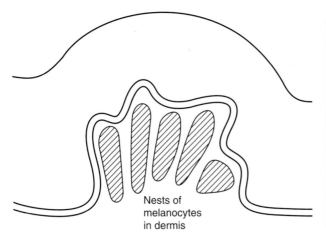

Figure 1.16 Diagrammatic representation of an intradermal melanocytic naevus.

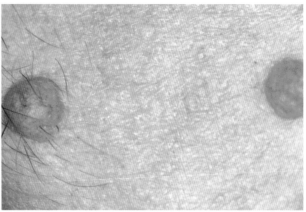

Figure 1.17 Intradermal melanocytic naevus.

Clinical features

The pigmented lesion suddenly develops a halo of depigmentation (Figure 1.18).

The central naevus gradually becomes smaller and eventually disappears. The remaining small area of hypopigmentation usually, but not always, slowly repigments over the next few months.

Management

The presence of the halo alone should not cause concern. Reassure the patient and explain the likely outcome. Review the patient every 6–8 weeks to reassure yourself and the patient that the lesion is behaving as expected.

There is no need to remove the pigmented lesion at the centre of the halo unless it behaves suspiciously. Should the naevus in the centre change in size, shape or colour it should be treated like any other suspicious pigmented lesion.

ATYPICAL MELANOCYTIC NAEVI

At least 5% of the population have one or two atypical melanocytic naevi, previously known as 'dysplastic naevi'. This term is no longer used because many clinicians associate dysplasia with inevitable malignant transformation.

Clinical features

Atypical naevi are large (usually 5 mm) with an irregular border, often variably pigmented, and sometimes have a pinkish inflammatory appearance (Figure 1.19). They are commonest on the trunk but also occur on the limbs.

Don't forget

The differential diagnosis is malignant melanoma.

Management

This is a difficult area where ideas are constantly changing. The confident diagnosis of an atypical naevus is not easy in general practice. Simple guidelines are as follows.

- **Solitary atypical melanocytic naevus:** The history can be helpful. If the atypical naevus has been present and unchanging for years it is unlikely to be a malignant melanoma. If the lesion is new or you are concerned about it, refer the patient for a dermatological opinion. It is very difficult to distinguish atypical melanocytic naevi clinically from *in situ* melanomas.
- **Multiple atypical melanocytic naevi:** A patient with many atypical naevi, particularly on unusual sites such as the scalp, buttocks or dorsum of the feet, should definitely see a dermatologist. The patient may have the atypical mole syndrome (Figure 1.20), which is associated with an increased incidence of malignant melanoma. It is most important to give this group of patients advice on sun avoidance and information about checking their moles for change in size, shape or colour.

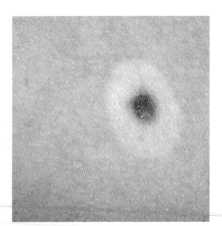

Figure 1.18 Halo naevus, also known as Sutton's naevus.

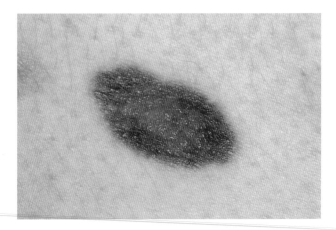

Figure 1.19 Atypical melanocytic naevus with an irregular border and variable pigmentation.

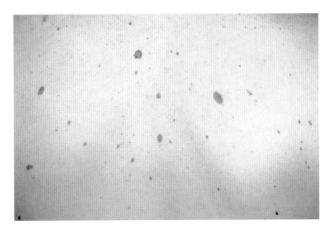

Figure 1.20   Multiple atypical melanocytic naevi in a patient with the atypical mole syndrome.

CONGENITAL MELANOCYTIC NAEVUS

These are melanocytic naevi which by definition are present at birth. Typically they are dark brown and may be raised, often having mamillary projections. Hair is often, but not always, present in varying amounts. Size is variable, but these naevi can be divided broadly into two groups:

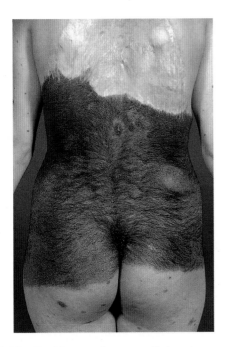

Figure 1.21   Bathing trunk congenital melanocytic naevus.

- Very extensive lesions covering large areas of the skin, such as the so-called bathing trunk or garment naevi (Figure 1.21). Fortunately, these are relatively rare. There is a definite increase in malignant transformation in these lesions.
- Small congenital naevi (Figure 1.22), which are relatively common and occur on any part of the body. Although there is evidence of a slightly increased risk of malignant change in these lesions, the risk has not yet been quantified.

Management

Patients with extensive congenital naevi should have long-term follow up, looking for malignant change.

Those with small congenital naevi should be advised to check them regularly for change in size, shape or colour. Any such change is an indication for referral.

Most dermatologists believe that, if a congenital naevus is small and would be easy to excise, it should be removed because of the slightly increased risk of malignant change

BLUE NAEVUS

This melanocytic lesion is less common than those already described.

Clinical features

A blue naevus typically appears in childhood or early adult life, most commonly on the extremities. It

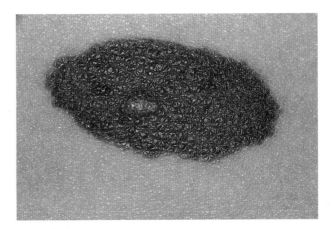

Figure 1.22   Small congenital melanocytic naevus. Congenital melanocytic naevi may resemble other types of pigmented melanocytic naevi but, by definition, are present at or shortly after birth.

is usually solitary, less than 1 cm in diameter, slightly raised and has a distinctive dark blue/slate grey colour (Figure 1.23).

Although the appearance is usually typical, it can sometimes resemble a malignant melanoma.

Management

If the clinical diagnosis is not in doubt and the lesion is unchanging, there is no need to remove it. If the diagnosis is in doubt or the lesion is changing, refer the patient to a specialist.

These lesions can be unsightly and patients may request excision for cosmetic reasons. Ellipse excision with a 2 mm margin is the best treatment, provided that the site is suitable.

SPITZ NAEVUS

Spitz naevus is a rare benign melanocytic lesion. The histological features may resemble malignant melanoma; hence the alternative term, 'juvenile melanoma', which is sometimes used by histopathologists.

Clinical features

Spitz naevi occur most commonly in young children but may be seen in young adults. The commonest site is the cheeks. The lesion typically presents as a rapidly enlarging red or reddish-brown nodule up to 1–2 cm in diameter (Figure 1.24).

The differential diagnosis includes pyogenic granuloma and, in young adults, malignant melanoma.

Management

If you suspect this diagnosis, refer the patient for a specialist to confirm the diagnosis. It will usually be necessary to excise the lesion for histological assessment. In the case of a young child this may require general anaesthesia. If the pathologist has any doubts about the histological diagnosis, wider excision may be necessary.

If you receive a histology report suggesting the diagnosis of Spitz naevus or juvenile melanoma, particularly when the patient is an adult, you should discuss the case with the histopathologist or dermatologist.

Basal cell papilloma (seborrhoeic keratosis)

Clinicians sometimes have difficulty with the terminology of these lesions. Seborrhoeic keratosis describes the clinical appearance, and basal cell papilloma the histological appearance of the lesion (Figure 1.25). Both are acceptable terms and can be used synonymously.

Senile keratosis, seborrhoeic wart and senile wart are terms best avoided. Many patients find the term 'senile' derogatory, and 'wart' suggests a viral aetiology, which may lead to the inappropriate use of antiviral wart preparations.

Clinical features

These pigmented lesions usually start to appear in the fifth decade. They occur equally in men and

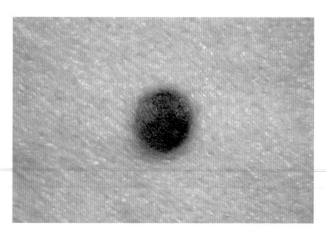

Figure 1.23 Blue naevus.

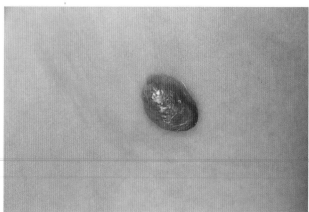

Figure 1.24 Clinical photograph of a Spitz naevus. This is rare and also known as juvenile melanoma.

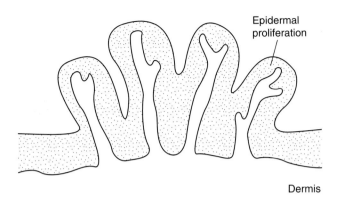

Figure 1.25 Diagrammatic representation of a basal cell papilloma (seborrhoeic keratosis).

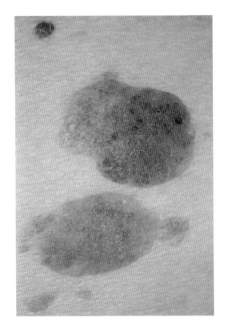

Figure 1.26 Basal cell papilloma (seborrhoeic keratosis).

women. They continue appearing in predisposed people for many years and do not resolve spontaneously. The elderly may have large areas of skin affected.

Seborrhoeic keratoses usually occur on the upper trunk and face. They are much commoner in white than in dark-skinned races. Usually ovoid, they vary in size from a few millimetres to 2–3 cm.

The lesion typically consists of a crusty, greasy (seborrhoeic) plaque, most of which is above the skin surface. It is adherent to the epidermis but looks as if it could be easily lifted off. The crusty surface often falls off only to re-form (Figures 1.26, 1.27).

The colour is variable but is most commonly black. Brownish yellow lesions also occur. They are often itchy and may become inflamed or 'irritated' when scratched. A diagnostic clue is the presence of plugged follicular orifices on the surface of the lesion, best seen using a hand lens.

Malignant change in basal cell papillomas is extremely rare and it is often said that it never occurs.

The differential diagnosis of basal cell papilloma is that of any pigmented lesion and includes benign melanocytic naevi and malignant melanoma. Indeed in many dermatology clinics the most commonly referred pigmented lesions suspected of being malignant melanoma are in fact basal cell papillomas.

Management

Explanation and reassurance are often all that is needed. Many people accept these lesions as a part of getting older. Where the diagnosis is certain and

the lesions are multiple it is important to tell the patient that new lesions are likely to continue appearing. You should avoid removing them in large numbers.

Some patients become very distressed by the unsightly appearance. In such cases it is important to help the patient come to terms with the problem. Some patients request treatment, and it is not unreasonable to remove basal cell papillomas that are symptomatic or disfiguring.

The correct way to remove basal cell papillomas is

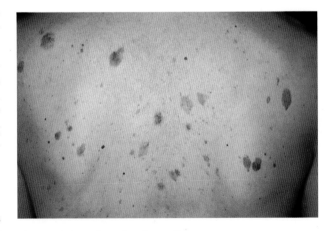

Figure 1.27 Basal cell papillomas are most commonly multiple.

by curettage and cautery (p. 115). Curettage leaves a flat surface, which rapidly re-epithelializes. Ellipse excision is not appropriate as it leaves an unjustifiable scar. However confident your diagnosis, always send the curettings for histological examination.

You may prefer to treat these lesions with cryotherapy (p. 120) but remember that this treatment does not provide you with histological confirmation, so you must be completely confident of your diagnosis.

Skin tag (fibro-epithelial polyp)

Clinical features

Skin tags are common and often occur in people with basal cell papillomas. These small, fleshy, pedunculated lesions are usually seen on the neck, in the flexures and around the eyes of the middle-aged and elderly (Figure 1.28).

Management

As with basal cell papillomas, new tags continue to appear in predisposed individuals. Skin tags are easy to remove by snip excision, with or without cautery. Some patients can be encouraged to snip them off themselves. Cotton can be tied round the base, but this can lead to swelling and an unpleasant inflammatory response and we do not recommend it.

Epidermoid cyst (pilar cyst)

This is best considered as a derivative of the pilosebaceous unit (Figure 1.29).

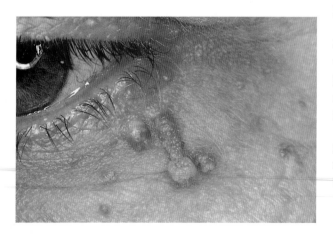

Figure 1.28 Skin tags.

Epidermoid cysts are often incorrectly referred to as 'sebaceous cysts'. True sebaceous cysts, which contain oily sebum, are actually very rare. An epidermoid cyst consists of an epidermoid wall surrounding a core containing keratin and its breakdown products. The contents have a characteristic semisolid, cheesy appearance and often a foul odour.

Clinical features

Epidermoid cysts are common in young and middle-aged adults, but rare in childhood. Teenagers with significant acne vulgaris are particularly prone to them. Epidermoid cysts are often asymptomatic. However they tend to enlarge slowly and sometimes become inflamed. The commonest sites are the head, neck, chest and back. They never occur on the palms or soles. The cysts may be single or multiple.

The spherical cyst is situated in the dermis. The overlying epidermis is normal and the cyst lifts this to a varying degree to give a domed appearance (Figure 1.30). In sites where there is little subcutaneous tissue, such as the scalp, the lesion is raised above the surrounding skin, causing the overlying epidermis to become taut. On the back, where it has room to expand into the subcutaneous tissue, the cyst is less likely to be raised. Often, but not always, a keratin-filled punctum may be seen, marking the point of attachment of the cyst to the epidermis.

Management

Many patients elect to have epidermoid cysts excised. Excision of a non-inflamed epidermoid cyst is usually straightforward and is the type of procedure that is very suitable to undertake in general practice. The technique is described in Chapter 7.

Don't forget

When the cyst is inflamed, the initial treatment is incision and drainage. If the residual cyst enlarges it may be removed electively when all the inflammation has resolved.

Cysts in areas of acne vulgaris are susceptible to recurrent inflammation and are often difficult to remove. They are best left until the acne has been treated effectively.

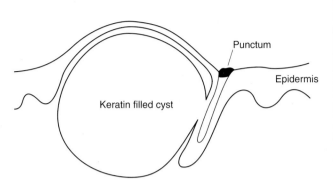

Figure 1.29 Diagrammatic representation of an epidermoid (pilar) cyst.

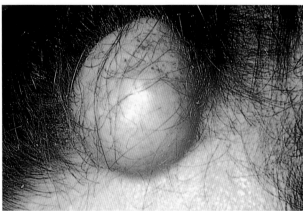

Figure 1.30 Epidermoid (pilar) cyst.

Dermatofibroma (histiocytoma)

This can be considered as a proliferation of fibroblasts in the dermis (Figure 1.31). It is generally accepted that it reflects an abnormal response to an insect bite, although a history of such a bite is obtained in only about 20% of those affected.

Clinical features

Dermatofibromas are common, particularly on the lower limbs of women. They usually present as a persistent, firm, hard nodule which is often itchy. The clinical appearances vary, depending upon the appearance of the overlying epidermis (Figure 1.32). Some are pigmented and may be confused with compound naevi.

Management

Where the clinical diagnosis is not in doubt there is no medical indication to excise dermatofibromas. Patients often request excision for cosmetic reasons. However you should select patients carefully because of the tendency of these lesions to occur on the lower limb. This is a bad area for healing and the resulting scar may look worse than the nodule you removed. Be sure to discuss fully with the patient the likely cosmetic outcome.

If you decide to proceed, ellipse excision is the appropriate procedure. We strongly recommend that the patient wears a support bandage until the sutures are removed, as with all procedures on the lower limb.

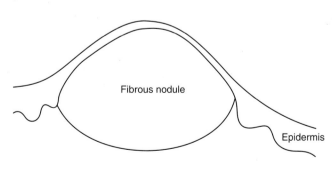

Figure 1.31 Diagrammatic representation of a dermatofibroma (histiocytoma).

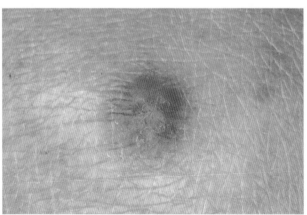

Figure 1.32 Typical example of a dermatofibroma (histiocytoma).

15

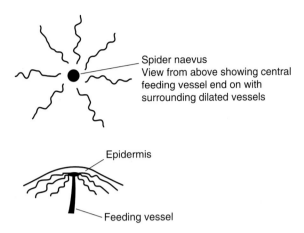

Figure 1.33 Diagrammatic representation of a spider naevus.

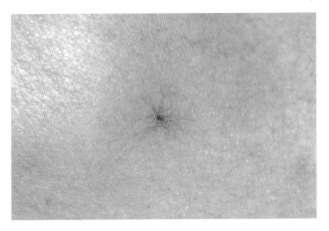

Figure 1.34 Spider naevus.

Angiomatous lesions

SPIDER NAEVI

These are small vascular malformations which usually occur on the face, neck, upper trunk and arms. They are common in women, particularly during pregnancy. Circulating oestrogens are thought to be relevant in the aetiology. A central dilated vessel is surrounded by numerous smaller vessels (Figures 1.33, 1.34). A useful diagnostic test is to press on the spider naevus with a glass microscope slide, which makes the lesion disappear.

Management

Many disappear spontaneously. Certainly those that develop during pregnancy usually resolve after delivery. Cold point electrocautery and the Hyfrecator can be used to coagulate the central vessel (p. 117). If you do not have the necessary equipment then you may choose to refer the patient to a dermatologist for treatment.

Don't forget

Although multiple spider naevi can be a feature of chronic liver disease, solitary spider naevi unrelated to liver disease are much more common.

CAMPBELL DE MORGAN SPOTS

These are caused by a benign proliferation of blood vessels high in the dermis, with overlying hyperkeratosis.

Clinical features

Campbell de Morgan spots are very common, particularly in the middle-aged and elderly. They are small, cherry-red spots, up to about 5 mm in diameter (Figure 1.35), and are usually multiple. They occur most commonly on the trunk. Excised lesions will be reported histologically as angiokeratomas.

Management

In view of the large numbers which may be present these are best left untreated. Patients should be warned that they are likely to develop new ones from time to time.

PYOGENIC GRANULOMA

Pyogenic granuloma is caused by a proliferation of blood vessels in the dermis (Figure 1.36).

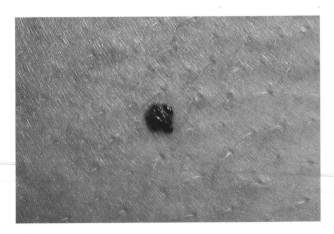

Figure 1.35 Campbell de Morgan spot.

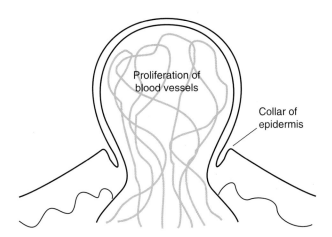

Figure 1.36 Diagrammatic representation of a pyogenic granuloma.

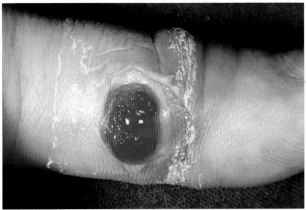

Figure 1.37 Pyogenic granuloma.

Clinical features

Pyogenic granulomas occur equally in both sexes and at any age. They are not uncommon in childhood. The commonest presentation is of a rapidly enlarging, juicy, non-pigmented lesion, usually on the extremities.

They are usually bright red and may be up to 10 mm in diameter (Figure 1.37). They bleed easily and profusely. Some patients give a history of a minor penetrating injury a few weeks before the development of the lesion.

Management

Pyogenic granulomas lend themselves well to curettage and cautery (Chapter 8), but be prepared for bleeding, which may be profuse. Although haemostasis can often be achieved by cautery it may be necessary to suture the skin after the lesion has been removed.

Don't forget

It is important to check that the histology report confirms the clinical diagnosis, as the most important differential diagnosis of a pyogenic granuloma is an amelanotic malignant melanoma (p. 28).

Viral warts

Clinical features

Warts are very common and management is often a problem for the clinician. They come in various shapes and sizes. Most are caused by infection with

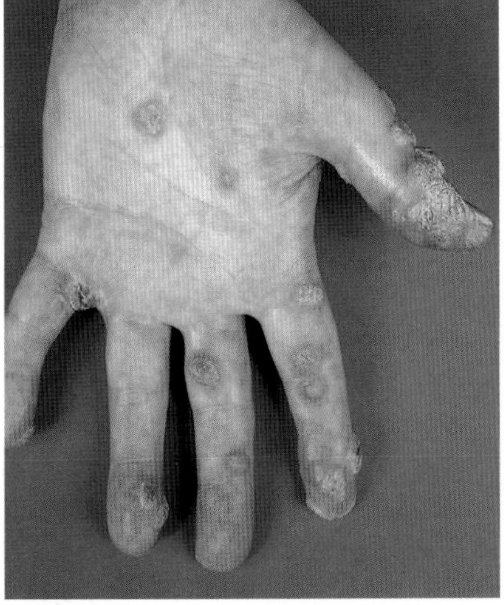

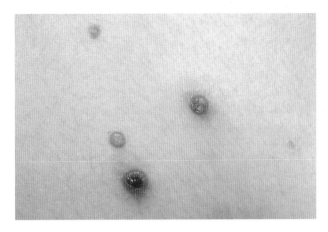

Figure 1.38 Digital warts.

Figure 1.39 Molluscum contagiosum.

17

Human papilloma virus (Figure 1.38). The exception is molluscum contagiosum, which is caused by pox virus (Figure 1.39).

The most important message about warts is that the vast majority will resolve spontaneously without scarring when the patient has developed an adequate immunological response. This may take months or years, during which time the patient may become fed up because of the cosmetic appearance. People with viral warts often ask to have them removed.

The temptation to remove warts surgically should be resisted wherever possible for the following reasons.

- Warts commonly recur at the site of surgical removal.
- The resulting scar is unnecessary, since the wart will eventually resolve without one.
- Curettage of large plantar warts inevitably leaves a large wound on the sole of the foot. This may be painful to walk on and the wart often recurs within the scar.
- Ellipse excision of warts leaves an inappropriate linear scar and warts may develop within this scar. This phenomenon is known as Köbnerization.
- Most warts occur in children, where unnecessary surgery should be avoided.
- Molluscum contagiosum can be very extensive, particularly in children, but the lesions usually resolve spontaneously without scarring in 6–9 months.
- The only possible exception might be filiform warts. These have a very narrow base and curettage, with or without cautery, will leave only a small scar. The wart may nevertheless recur!

Accepted treatments

- **Time:** Most warts resolve spontaneously in 3–6 months. The evaluation of any treatment method has to take this into account.
- **Keratolytic wart paints:** There are many products, usually containing salicylic and lactic acid. These need to be used every night for up to 3 months. The patient should be instructed to soak the area in water. After drying, the hard skin should be pared down using a pumice stone or emery board. Finally the preparation is applied. The newer gels avoid the need to protect the surrounding normal skin and to wear an occlusive dressing.

- **Formaldehyde soaks:** This rather old-fashioned method is undoubtedly effective for many plantar warts. A litre of 3% formaldehyde is supplied to the patient. The affected foot is soaked in a bowl of the solution for 15 minutes each evening. Warn the patient to use an old bowl. The solution is poured back into the bottle each evening (using a funnel) and can be reused. Because of evaporation it is necessary to top up the bottle from time to time with water.
- **Liquid nitrogen cryotherapy:** Details of this procedure are to be found in Chapter 8. For cryotherapy to be effective it must cause tissue destruction. This is inevitably painful and should therefore be avoided in children. Adequate cryotherapy to plantar warts may leave the patient unable to walk for several days after the treatment.

Chondrodermatitis nodularis helicis

Chondrodermatitis nodularis helicis is a benign condition of inflammation of the cartilage of the pinna, with overlying dermal and epidermal inflammation. It is quite common and the diagnosis is usually straightforward. It can be very rewarding to treat.

Clinical features

The condition usually occurs in men over the age of 40, although women are also affected. Although other parts of the pinna can be involved, the patient typically presents with a very painful and exquisitely tender inflamed nodule (0.5–1.0 cm in diameter)

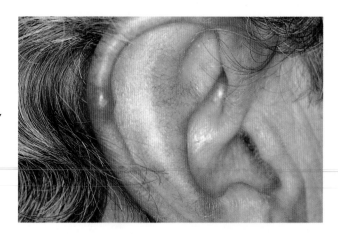

Figure 1.40 Chondrodermatitis nodularis helicis.

at the upper pole of the helix (Figure 1.40). The condition usually occurs on the side on which the patient sleeps, and the severe pain often interferes with sleeping.

Management

It is important to try some simple measures to relieve pressure on the helix while awaiting surgery. Corn plasters can be used, cutting out a central disc the size of the nodule.

Surgical excision of the lesion with a margin of normal skin is the treatment of choice. If the lesion is small you may feel happy to do this yourself; otherwise refer the patient to a dermatologist or surgeon.

Although the extreme tenderness of the lesion usually makes the diagnosis straightforward, remember that squamous cell carcinoma on the pinna can sometimes mimic chondrodermatitis nodularis helicis, and vice versa.

PREMALIGNANT SKIN LESIONS

This section considers solar keratoses, Bowen's disease, keratoacanthomas and Hutchinson's freckle (lentigo maligna). While not truly benign, these conditions are not quite malignant. It is important to try to make a firm clinical diagnosis of these lesions, as simple excision is often not the most appropriate treatment.

Solar keratoses are common on the sun-damaged skin of the elderly. Their association with the development of squamous cell carcinoma is not clear-cut, and spontaneous resolution of solar keratoses often occurs. Bowen's disease and keratoacanthomas are relatively uncommon. Bowen's disease will definitely progress to squamous cell carcinoma if left for long enough. Keratoacanthomas demonstrate many of the clinical and histological features of malignancy, but they behave very differently. Hutchinson's freckle (lentigo maligna) is becoming commoner and if left will progress to invasive lentigo maligna melanoma.

Solar keratosis (actinic keratosis, senile keratosis)

Solar keratoses are common on the light-exposed skin of fair-skinned people who have had a large amount of cumulative sun exposure. The relationship between sunlight and the development of solar keratoses is well documented, and these lesions are particularly common in white Australians. There is debate about the likelihood of malignant change but it is generally accepted that the risk of transformation is very small. Remember that the presence of one or two of these lesions is evidence that the patient has had long periods of sun exposure and is at risk of developing further solar keratoses, as well as tumours associated with chronic sun exposure.

Clinical features

The characteristic appearance is that of a pink, scaly, warty or crusted lesion on the face, scalp, ears and backs of the hands (Figure 1.41). Sometimes a solar keratosis may present as a cutaneous horn (Figure 1.42).

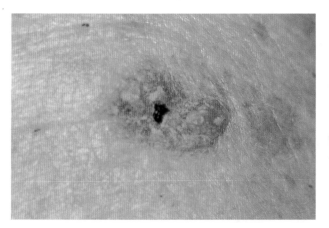

Figure 1.41 Solar (actinic) keratosis.

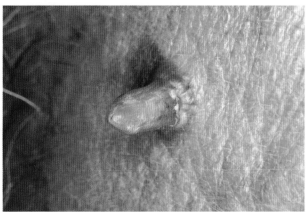

Figure 1.42 Solar keratosis presenting as a cutaneous horn.

Lesions are often multiple (Figure 1.43) and are frequently more obvious in the summer.

Patients will often report that some of their keratoses regress spontaneously in the winter. Solar keratoses are usually no more than a cosmetic nuisance. They are usually asymptomatic, although they may occasionally itch.

Malignant transformation of a solar keratosis is rare but is suggested by induration at the base and an increase in the inflammatory change around the lesion. The appearance of a nodule within the lesion is also suspicious. Squamous cell carcinoma arising in a solar keratosis is usually, but not always, slowly growing, with little tendency to metastasize.

Management

Since these lesions regress when sunlight is avoided, a sunscreen and protective clothing (e.g. a hat) should be used. This will also prevent the development of new lesions.

- **Solitary lesions:**
  - *Cryotherapy:* If the patient is keen to have the solar keratosis removed, liquid nitrogen is the treatment of choice, provided that the clinical diagnosis is not in doubt and histological confirmation is not required. The cosmetic result is usually good but patients should be warned of the short-term effects of treatment and of the long-term possibility of developing a hypopigmented macule (p. 120).
  - *Curettage and cautery:* This is an effective treatment, with the additional benefit that the curettings can be sent for histological examination. However this is even more likely than cryotherapy to leave superficial scarring which may make the treatment unjustifiable (p. 115).
  - *5-fluorouracil:* Some dermatologists cautiously use 5-fluorouracil. This is an aggressive topical anti-mitotic agent which may cause nasty ulceration during treatment. Experience of the drug's effect is required to use it safely and effectively, and this treatment is not recommended for use in general practice.
- **Multiple lesions:** Treatment is more difficult when the lesions are multiple. Repeated cryotherapy or curettage and cautery should be avoided as unacceptable scarring may result. Patients who request treatment for multiple lesions, or in whom there is concern about malignant transformation, should be referred to a dermatologist.

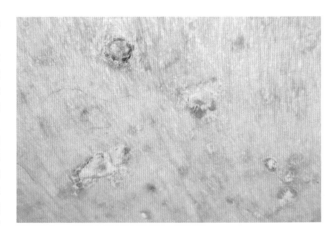

Figure 1.43 Solar (actinic) keratoses are commonly multiple.

Bowen's disease (intra-epidermal squamous cell carcinoma)

Bowen's disease is much rarer than solar keratosis and represents a skin tumour that has progressed one stage closer to the development of squamous cell carcinoma. Also known as intra-epidermal carcinoma *in situ*, it inevitably progresses to squamous cell carcinoma, although this may take many years. Spontaneous resolution does not occur. There is an association between cumulative sun exposure and Bowen's disease, though this is less clear-cut than with solar keratosis. Ingestion or topical application of arsenical preparations (e.g. tonics, Fowler's solution) is known to predispose to the development of this condition.

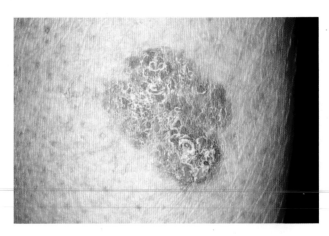

Figure 1.44 Patch of Bowen's disease on the lower limb.

Clinical features

Bowen's disease presents as a persistent, well-demarcated, erythematous, scaly plaque on the lower limb of the elderly. The plaque enlarges and may reach several centimetres in diameter (Figure 1.44).

Differential diagnosis

This includes inflammatory dermatoses such as psoriasis, tinea corporis and discoid eczema. Treatment with topical steroids or antifungals is, however, ineffective. If ulceration or a nodule develops within the lesion, malignant change should be suspected.

Management

Since the tumour most commonly occurs on the lower limbs of the elderly, where healing after surgery is often poor, primary surgical excision is usually inappropriate, particularly if the lesion is large.

Where Bowen's disease is strongly suspected clinically, and the patient is reluctant or too frail to be referred to hospital, histological confirmation of the diagnosis can be obtained by taking a small incision biopsy from the centre of the lesion.

The most widely used treatment is liquid nitrogen cryotherapy. If the lesion is large it should be treated in stages, ensuring that healing has occurred before proceeding to the next part of the plaque. A reasonable interval between treatments would be 4–6 weeks.

The risk of progression to squamous cell carcinoma should not be underestimated, and you should only embark on treating Bowen's disease if you fully understand the potential problems.

Keratoacanthoma

This is a spontaneously resolving tumour that is much less common than either solar keratosis or Bowen's disease. Keratoacanthoma occurs at about a third of the frequency of squamous cell carcinoma, which is the most important clinical and histological differential diagnosis. It is often difficult to distinguish between the two conditions, particularly histologically. Again there seems to be a link with sun exposure, since keratoacanthomas are most commonly seen on the head or upper limb of the middle-aged and elderly.

Clinical features

A keratoacanthoma is usually a solitary lesion that enlarges rapidly over 4–12 weeks, causing considerable alarm to some patients.

The typical lesion is a neatly symmetrical pink nodule 10–20 mm in diameter, and has a central crater filled with a keratin plug (Figures 1.45, 1.46).

Occasionally the tumour may be as large as 50 mm in diameter. The surrounding skin is often normal, with a marked absence of the thickening and induration that occurs around a nodule of squamous cell carcinoma. Left alone, spontaneous resolution occurs within about 3 months. The diagnostic

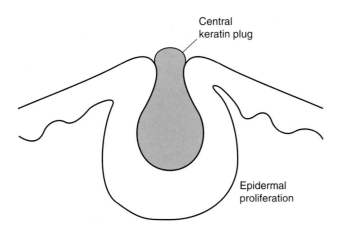

Figure 1.45 Diagrammatic representation of a keratoacanthoma.

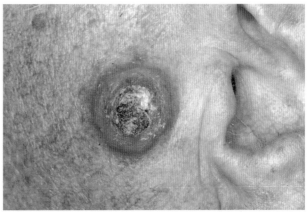

Figure 1.46 Typical keratoacanthoma. Note the symmetry of the lesion and the central keratin-filled crater.

21

clues suggesting keratoacanthoma are the short history and the tidy symmetrical appearance of the lesion.

Management

Despite the tendency to resolution the treatment of choice is urgent excision. The important differential diagnosis is a rapidly enlarging squamous cell carcinoma. It is therefore vital that the specimen is sent for careful histological examination.

The histopathology report itself may cause some difficulty. It will often state that the diagnosis of squamous cell carcinoma cannot be excluded histologically and that the history and clinical appearances of the lesion should be taken into consideration when deciding on the definitive diagnosis and further management.

In view of the potential pitfalls it is more appropriate to refer patients with lesions suggestive of keratoacanthoma to a dermatologist for assessment and surgery. The clinical appearance of the tumour is vital in making a correct diagnosis. Provided the tumour has been completely excised, then the outcome is likely to be satisfactory (p. 39).

Hutchinson's freckle (lentigo maligna)

This represents a proliferation of atypical melanocytes that is premalignant. Although much less common than solar keratosis and Bowen's disease, Hutchinson's freckle is not rare and is becoming more common as people live longer. Again, cumulative sun exposure is the important aetiological factor.

Clinical features

This is a slowly enlarging pigmented lesion which occurs on the face, upper cheek, temple or forehead of the elderly. Initially it appears as a flat brown mark which then gradually enlarges and becomes darker, usually with variation in colour (Figure 1.47) and an irregular border. By the time the patient presents, the lesion may be quite large (2 cm diameter).

The lesion with which it is most commonly confused is a basal cell papilloma. The smoothness of the skin and absence of the typical warty texture of a basal cell papilloma can be useful clues to support the diagnosis of a Hutchinson's freckle. The uniform pigmentation of the basal cell papilloma or solar lentigo contrasts sharply with the variable pigmentation of Hutchinson's freckle.

After slowly enlarging over a period of some years, a nodule may develop. This indicates transformation into an invasive lentigo maligna melanoma, which has a poor prognosis for survival.

Management

If you suspect a Hutchinson's freckle you should refer the patient to a specialist. Multiple biopsies of suspicious areas may be necessary to confirm the diagnosis. Following histological confirmation, complete excision of the affected area is necessary, often with skin grafting.

Always look very carefully at brown patches on the face of the elderly and consider the diagnosis of Hutchinson's freckle. Treatment prevents the development of invasive lentigo maligna melanoma.

MALIGNANT SKIN LESIONS

Malignant skin lesions are much less common than benign ones. The aim of this section is to describe the clinical features of the commoner skin malignancies. Think carefully before excising skin malignancies in general practice. Although these tumours are often fairly easy to remove, it is more difficult to make an accurate preoperative diagnosis because they are so uncommon. If you do decide to remove a lesion that may be malignant, you must have a clear management plan. You must have a clear idea of how you will proceed and what you will tell the patient when you receive the histology report. Remember that if you are uncertain about the clinical diagnosis you should not perform the surgery yourself.

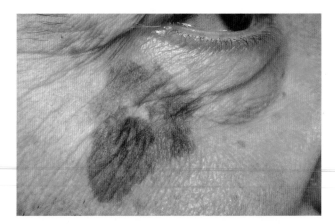

Figure 1.47 Hutchinson's freckle, also known as lentigo maligna.

Classification

Skin cancer can be divided into melanoma and non-melanoma skin cancer (Table 1.2).

This is a very important distinction. Non-melanoma skin cancer is common, for the most part slow growing, locally invasive and usually easily treatable. Melanoma skin cancer is much less common, more aggressive and will metastasize if not treated early. This distinction is important when counselling patients, many of whom think 'skin cancer, no hope'. This is because they have heard only about the depressingly poor prognosis for patients with malignant melanoma in the past.

Non-melanoma skin cancer

BASAL CELL CARCINOMA (RODENT ULCER)

Basal cell carcinoma (BCC), also known as rodent ulcer, is the commonest type of skin cancer in white-skinned people. This tumour is much commoner than the other malignant or premalignant tumours discussed in this chapter. Indeed, it is the commonest form of malignant disease.

BCCs enlarge very slowly but can be highly invasive locally. They are said not to metastasize. The commonest sites are the sun-damaged skin of the head and neck, especially in elderly patients who have had long periods of sun exposure over many years. The growing popularity of sunbathing has resulted in an increased incidence of these tumours in younger people.

Clinical features

- **Nodulocystic BCC:** This is the commonest type and usually appears on the face as a slowly enlarging nodule with a cystic, pearly appearance. It is often crossed by telangiectatic vessels (Figure 1.48). The nodule typically has a rolled edge and the patient often presents with a non-healing ulcer (Figure 1.49). In the past, these tumours caused extensive destruction of large areas of the face, hence the name rodent ulcer.

Other types listed below are variants of a typical basal cell carcinoma and are much less common:
- **Pigmented BCC:** Sometimes a BCC is pigmented (Figure 1.50), causing confusion with a melanoma.
- **Superficial BCC:** Unlike the other types, superficial BCCs are usually seen on the trunk. Cystic change is usually seen at the periphery of the

Table 1.2 Melanoma and non-melanoma skin cancer: the differences

Non-melanoma skin cancer	Melanoma skin cancer
Basal cell carcinoma, squamous cell carcinoma	Malignant melanoma
Common	Much less common
Older (50 years upwards)	Younger (30–70, mean 51 years)
Sun-exposed sites, weathered skin	Commoner on legs in women and trunk in men
Slowly enlarging	More rapidly enlarging
Locally invasive	
Metastases from basal cell carcinomas virtually unheard of	Metastasizes early
Squamous cell carcinomas may metastasize, usually at a late stage	
Prognosis for survival excellent	Prognosis for survival excellent if diagnosed early; terrible if diagnosed late
Second tumours common	

lesion. The differential diagnosis includes Bowen's disease and inflammatory dermatoses such as eczema, psoriasis and tinea corporis (Figure 1.51). As with Bowen's disease, treatment with topical steroids or antifungals will be ineffective.

- **Morphoeic BCC:** This is the least common type, which is fortunate since it is the most difficult to diagnose and treat (Figure 1.52). The affected area is often thickened and pale, and the typical cystic change with telangiectasia may be absent.

Differential diagnosis

To the inexperienced (and experienced!) eye, sebaceous gland hyperplasia (Figure 1.53) and non-pigmented intradermal naevi may be difficult to distinguish from basal cell carcinoma. If there is any doubt the patient should be referred for a further opinion, to avoid unnecessary surgery.

Management

- **Nodulocystic BCC:** The treatment of choice is surgical excision. Radiotherapy is still sometimes appropriate, although the resulting scar is much worse. Curettage and cautery has been advocated and this technique works well for some patients, but it should only be performed by clinicians with a sound dermatological training and expertise in the diagnosis and management of skin tumours. Curettings should always be sent for histological

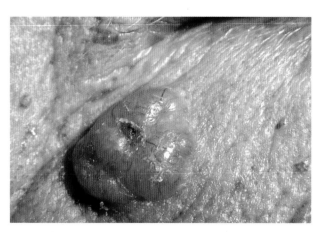

Figure 1.48 Nodulocystic basal cell carcinoma.

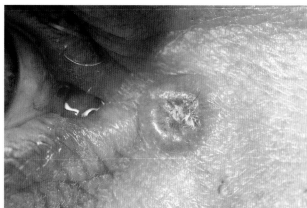

Figure 1.49 Many nodulocystic basal cell carcinomas present as a non-healing ulcer.

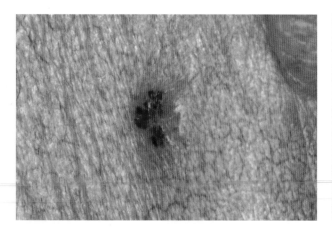

Figure 1.50 Pigmented basal cell carcinomas can sometimes be difficult to distinguish from malignant melanoma.

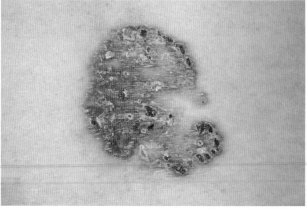

Figure 1.51 Superficial basal cell carcinoma. These are commonly seen on the trunk, unlike nodular basal cell carcinomas which are usually on the head and neck.

examination. Diagnostic biopsy of BCCs is of little value if the patient is to be referred for definitive surgery anyway.

- **Morphoeic BCC:** Clinically these tumours have a very poorly defined margin. They may require a procedure known as Moh's micrographic surgery. This is usually performed by a dermatological surgeon in close collaboration with a histopathologist. A primary excision is performed and, with the patient still in the operating theatre, frozen sections of the specimen are examined to establish if the tumour has been fully excised. Further excision can be performed as necessary and the process repeated until the tumour has been completely removed.
- **Superficial BCC:** These are the only BCCs for which liquid nitrogen cryotherapy is indicated and they usually respond well to this treatment.

Where a confident clinical diagnosis of BCC has been made in a frail, elderly patient, excision in the GP's surgery may be more convenient. Provided the specimen is sent for histological examination and the lesion is completely excised, both patient and surgeon can be satisfied with the outcome.

Recurrence may take some years to develop so the patient should be reviewed at intervals and be advised to return if the scar changes, even after a very long time. Second tumours are common, with 20% of patients developing a second BCC within 5 years. It is therefore important to check the rest of the skin of a patient presenting with a BCC. Further advice about follow-up is discussed in Chapter 3.

SQUAMOUS CELL CARCINOMA (EPITHELIOMA)

Squamous cell carcinoma (SCC, epithelioma) typically arises in the sun-damaged skin of the elderly. It is much less common than basal cell carcinoma. Since it is more aggressive, correct diagnosis and management are vital. The tumour can arise *de novo*, or there may be a history of a preceding long-standing solar keratosis or a patch of Bowen's disease.

Clinical features

The commonest early clinical presentation is of an indurated crusted keratotic plaque or nodule (Figure 1.54). Later, a non-healing ulcer may develop, with an irregular raised border (Figure 1.55).

The rate of enlargement is variable but it is usually faster than that of basal cell carcinomas and slower than that of keratoacanthomas. Squamous cell carcinomas do metastasize, although tumours arising in solar keratoses are particularly slow to do so. Lesions on the lip spread earlier and have a worse prognosis.

Differential diagnosis

Keratoacanthoma is the most difficult differential diagnosis. Even if the clinical diagnosis is keratoacanthoma, the histology report is often suggestive of a squamous cell carcinoma. It is very important to follow such patients up even if the lesion was completely removed (p. 39).

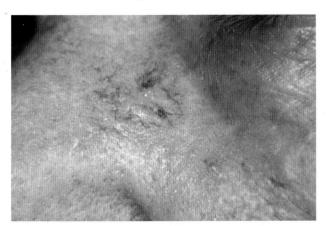

Figure 1.52 Morphoeic basal cell carcinoma. These lesions are often poorly defined and difficult to treat.

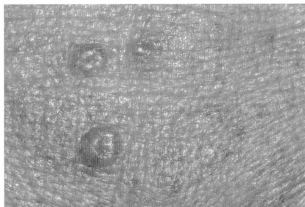

Figure 1.53 Sebaceous gland hyperplasia.

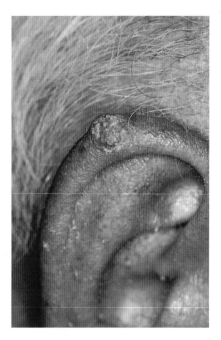

Figure 1.54 Small infiltrated keratotic nodule of squamous cell carcinoma.

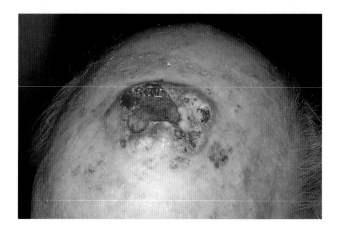

Figure 1.55 Large squamous cell carcinoma.

Management

This depends on the clinical presentation, site and, most importantly, the histopathological features. If the diagnosis of squamous cell carcinoma is suspected it is advisable to seek a specialist opinion before proceeding, since the combined expertise of a dermatologist, plastic surgeon and radiotherapist may be necessary. If a squamous cell carcinoma is excised unexpectedly you should refer the patient to a dermatologist for further assessment, histology review and development of a management plan appropriate to the aggressiveness of the tumour. Small tumours arising in actinic keratoses often do well with local excision alone, while larger, more aggressive tumours may require excision and radiotherapy. Occasionally, radiotherapy alone is indicated.

Malignant melanoma

Although the incidence of malignant melanoma has doubled in the last 10 years, this tumour is much less common than other types of skin cancer. An average general practitioner in the UK will probably see only one every 10 years. The prognosis of malignant melanoma is excellent if diagnosed and treated early, but remains poor if the tumour is diagnosed late.

Excision of melanoma in primary care

Whenever you examine a pigmented lesion you should ask yourself 'Could this be a malignant melanoma?'

There are two possible scenarios. In the first you suspect when you first see the patient that the lesion may be a malignant melanoma. In the second you excise a malignant melanoma inadvertently, only finding out when you receive the histopathology report.

- **You suspect the lesion is a malignant melanoma:** Although you may have the technical expertise for primary surgical excision of a malignant melanoma you should **not** undertake this in general practice.

  Because of the rarity of the tumour you cannot be expected to have up-to-date knowledge about the management and prognosis of patients with malignant melanoma.

  When you receive the histopathology report it is unlikely that you will be confident in counselling your patient and answering questions accurately. If a wider excision is required the patient will need to be referred to a specialist anyway. All dermatologists should agree to see a patient urgently (within a week) if you consider the diagnosis to be a malignant melanoma.

- **It looked benign but the histopathologist reports it as a malignant melanoma:** Do not panic! Do not immediately phone the patient. Take advice. Discuss the histopathology report urgently with your local dermatologist or plastic surgeon. It is most helpful if you can read the histology report out verbatim. Having taken advice about how to proceed, contact the patient. Provided you act promptly you will have done no harm to your patient. Even if you have carried out an incomplete excision of a melanoma, this is no worse than an incision biopsy. The old wives' tale about 'interfering with moles making them go bad' is not true.

Table 1.3 Pigmented lesions: the major and minor criteria

Major criteria	Minor criteria
Change in size	Inflammation
Change in shape	Crusting or bleeding
Change in colour	Sensory change
	Diameter greater than 7 mm

Natural history

Malignant melanoma affects young adults, and females are affected twice as commonly as males. The tumour is commoner in those who burn rather than tan in the sun. The history is of great importance since in many cases it forms the basis on which a decision to excise a pigmented lesion will be taken. Remember that in 70% of cases, malignant melanoma presents as a new mole, and in the remainder it occurs in a pre-existing naevus. A new enlarging pigmented lesion on the leg of a red-headed young woman should ring alarm bells even if it looks innocent at first glance.

Retrospective studies of patients with malignant melanoma have shown that the three most important worrying clinical signs in a pigmented naevus are **change in size, shape or colour.** These are the so-called major criteria. Symptoms such as itching are much less important and are included in the minor criteria (Table 1.3).

Clinical features

The commonest type of malignant melanoma is the superficial spreading type (80%). Invasive lentigo maligna melanoma is a condition of the elderly and is likely to become more common as people live longer. The other types (nodular, acral lentiginous and subungual) are rare and further information about them can be obtained from any standard dermatology text.

- **Superficial spreading malignant melanoma:** This is commonest on the legs of women and the trunk of men. It is a pigmented lesion, usually greater than 7 mm in diameter and often with an irregular

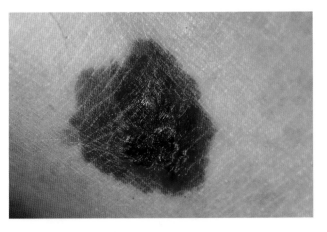

Figure 1.56 Superficial spreading malignant melanoma. This is by far the commonest type of malignant melanoma.

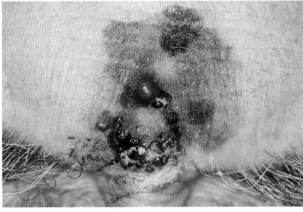

Figure 1.57 Invasive lentigo maligna melanoma arising in a long-standing Hutchinson's freckle (lentigo maligna).

border (Figure 1.56). The pigmentation within the lesion is variable and in some parts may even be absent.

- **Lentigo maligna melanoma:** The development of a nodule in a long-standing Hutchinson's freckle (lentigo maligna) indicates the development of invasive lentigo maligna melanoma (Figure 1.57).
- **Amelanotic malignant melanoma:** Although this is a very rare type of malignant melanoma, it is worth mentioning briefly. An amelanotic malignant melanoma typically presents as a rapidly enlarging shiny red nodule which may resemble the much commoner pyogenic granuloma (p. 16). The presence of a pre-existing pigmented lesion in which the nodule has developed is strongly suggestive of an amelanotic malignant melanoma. Because of the clinical similarity between the two lesions, all pyogenic granulomas should be excised urgently and the histology report should be checked carefully.

Prognosis of malignant melanoma

The single most important prognostic factor in malignant melanoma is the thickness of the tumour, the so-called Breslow thickness (Figure 1.58).

Excision of early lesions, which are thin (less than 1.5 mm), is associated with 90% 5-year survival. If the tumour is 1.5–3.5 mm in thickness, 5-year survival is around 70%, and if it is greater than 3.5 mm this figure falls to only 40%.

Management

Treatment of malignant melanoma remains surgical since the tumour is unresponsive to either chemotherapy or radiotherapy. The extensive mutilating surgery performed previously is now felt to be inappropriate. Ideally a malignant melanoma that is less than 2 mm in thickness should be excised with a 1 cm margin. A management plan for patients with thicker, poorer-prognosis tumours is usually agreed between plastic surgeons and dermatologists.

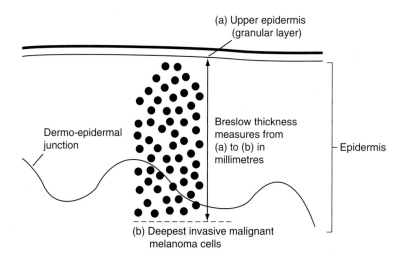

Figure 1.58 Measuring the Breslow thickness.

Chapter 2
Management: basic principles and clinical confusions

BASIC PRINCIPLES

It is not necessary to remove a lesion just because it is there. The right treatment for many lesions is to do nothing, and many patients only need reassurance.

> *Golden rule: never remove any lesion without a diagnosis.*

In many cases you will be able to make a confident clinical diagnosis. Chapter 1 contains an outline of the different treatments that are available and recommendations on those most suitable for particular conditions. Not infrequently a patient will present with a lesion you cannot identify; nevertheless you can usually decide if it is benign or malignant.

> *Golden rule: take a careful history.*

The history usually gives you the answer. A lesion that has been present for a long time and is not changing is almost certainly benign. However various points in the history may make you suspect malignant change.

For example, malignant change is suggested by a history of:
- change in size, shape or colour in a pre-existing melanocytic naevus;
- a new melanocytic lesion in a patient over the age of 40, particularly where it is rapidly enlarging, has an irregular outline or is variable in colour;
- development of a nodule in a pigmented patch on the face. This suggests development of invasive malignant melanoma in a Hutchinson's freckle.

Non-melanoma skin cancer is suggested by:
- a slowly enlarging, non-healing lesion on light-exposed skin (basal cell carcinoma);
- thickening, ulceration or nodule formation in a previously stable solar keratosis (squamous cell carcinoma);
- a nodule arising on an erythematous plaque on the leg, which may be a squamous cell carcinoma arising in a patch of Bowen's disease;
- any new, enlarging lesion on the skin of the elderly (squamous cell carcinoma, basal cell carcinoma).

Itching alone is not usually a symptom of malignancy. However, in combination with other symptoms it should be taken more seriously.

If you can identify the lesion

If you can make a diagnosis it is fairly straightforward to decide what to do next.

IF OBVIOUSLY BENIGN

Patients request removal of a lesion because it is a nuisance, it is unsightly or they are worried that it might be something sinister.

Should you remove it?

Ask yourself if there is any reason for the lesion to be removed. Many benign lesions are best treated with reassurance; to tamper with these is unnecessary and meddlesome.

Can you remove it?

In the case of a benign lesion you must decide if your skill, experience and facilities are adequate to deal with it. You should be certain that you can produce a result that will be better than the original lesion. Although no one expects you to be an expert plastic surgeon, you need to weigh up the potential problems against your skills in dealing with them and decide each case on its merits. The site of a lesion, its size and your own experience should all be considered.

There are a number of anatomical areas that should be avoided (Chapter 6). In addition, you should steer clear of surgery in certain groups of patients such as young children, very anxious patients and the litigiously inclined. It goes without saying that you must send any lesion you remove for histological examination. Sometimes you will get a surprise when the report comes back, and occasionally a nasty shock such as a completely unexpected malignancy. Chapter 3 deals with what to do if this happens.

IF OBVIOUSLY MALIGNANT

Sometimes you will suspect strongly that a lesion is malignant.

Pigmented lesion

The worry is that it may be a malignant melanoma. This needs prompt action. **Do not remove the lesion yourself but refer the patient at once.** Telephone your local consultant dermatologist and arrange for your patient to be seen within a week.

Non-pigmented lesion

Usually you will suspect either a basal cell (BCC) or a squamous cell carcinoma (SCC). Unless you have particular experience of treating patients with such lesions they should all be referred. Write to your local dermatologist, marking your letter 'Urgent'. They should preferably be seen at the dermatology clinic within 2–4 weeks. A suspected SCC needs to be seen sooner than a suspected BCC.

If you cannot identify the lesion

IF OBVIOUSLY BENIGN

Even if you cannot make a definite diagnosis you can often be sure that a lesion is harmless. Patients with such lesions do not have to be referred. If the lesion is stable, unchanging and has no sinister features you may well feel able to reassure your patient that nothing further needs to be done. You should always provide a safety net, however, by telling patients to see you again if they are at all concerned in the future.

Sometimes you may not be entirely happy with this approach. You may feel that there are features you are unsure about or that your patient has not been fully reassured. In this case arrange to review the patient after 6–12 weeks. There is little point in seeing him or her much sooner than 6 weeks, as little will have changed.

It is useful to draw a diagram of the lesion and to measure it in order to monitor any change in shape or size. If, when you review your patient, the lesion has not altered at all, you can reassure him or her strongly. Nevertheless, you should always tell the patient to consult you in the future if the lesion changes or if he or she at all worried. If you are unhappy in any way, refer for a specialist opinion at this stage.

IF POSSIBLY MALIGNANT

If you are not confident that the lesion is benign, you should refer the patient at this stage. Any change in size, shape or colour of a lesion is significant, and such a history should ring warning bells. Itching is a highly unreliable sign, although patients are often alarmed by it. Obviously you should have a low threshold for referring pigmented lesions, which can be very difficult to assess. **Always err on the side of caution.**

RASHES

It is an understandable temptation to biopsy rashes, in order to spare the patient a visit to hospital. In general you should resist the temptation, as there are dangers, not least a dissatisfied patient!

- **Wrong site:** You may take the biopsy from the wrong site. The report you receive will show non-specific changes and you are bound to refer the patient. The first biopsy will have resulted in a delay in diagnosis and treatment. If there is diagnostic doubt a further biopsy may be necessary and the patient may perceive the first one as having been inappropriate.

- **Incomprehensible report:** You may take a good biopsy from the correct site but receive an incomprehensible histopathology report. You will have to refer the patient anyway for the dermatologist to see the rash that goes with the report. The biopsy will have caused delay in treatment and the patient may have suffered undue anxiety.
- **Missed pathology:** In the worst scenario the biopsy misses the pathological features completely, giving false reassurance to the patient and doctor. The clinician at best misses a treatable condition and at worst misses a serious underlying disorder, e.g. cutaneous lymphoma.
- **Unnecessary biopsy:** Is a biopsy really necessary? Dermatologists look at lots of rashes and will often diagnose and start treatment without needing a biopsy at all.

Summary

Manage it yourself if:
- confident of benign diagnosis
- it needs no treatment
- it needs treatment and you can do it yourself
- it needs observation to reassure you and your patient.

Refer if:
- definitely malignant
- suspicious
- benign but needs treatment that is beyond your ability
- undiagnosed rash
- in any doubt about management.

COMMON CLINICAL CONFUSIONS

Introduction

There will be situations when you are unsure about the diagnosis of a skin lesion. Where the lesions in the differential diagnosis are all benign and their management is similar, being unable to make a correct diagnosis is irritating to the doctor but causes no harm to the patient. There are situations, however, even with benign lesions, when making the wrong diagnosis may lead to serious errors in management.

DIAGNOSIS WRONG, LESION BENIGN, ACCEPTABLE PROCEDURE PERFORMED

Sometimes a solar keratosis is thought to be a basal cell papilloma and is treated either by cryotherapy or curettage and cautery. Provided that the patient was keen to have the lesion treated and the lesion was definitely benign no harm has been done.

Epidermoid cysts and dermatofibromas are often confused. Here the correct diagnosis becomes clear during the surgical procedure, when a well-demarcated cyst rather than a fibrous dermal nodule is discovered, or vice versa. The outcome in both cases is a linear scar and provided the patient has requested the excision no harm will have been done.

DIAGNOSIS WRONG, LESION BENIGN, UNACCEPTABLE PROCEDURE PERFORMED

By far the commonest example of this is where a basal cell papilloma is incorrectly diagnosed as a benign melanocytic naevus and is removed by ellipse excision, leaving a sutured linear scar. This procedure is inappropriate and the patient will have reason to be dissatisfied with your management. The correct procedure is curettage and cautery, which leads to a much better cosmetic result (p. 115).

DIAGNOSIS WRONG, LESION MALIGNANT

This is the most worrying situation because incorrect diagnosis can lead to inappropriate management and the patient's care may suffer in consequence.

Examples of clinical confusions

MALIGNANT MELANOMA VERSUS BASAL CELL PAPILLOMA

These lesions are often mistaken for one another. Increase in size and change in colour, major criteria for the diagnosis of melanoma, are often the presenting features in both (p. 27). The lesion in Figure 2.1, despite its suspiciously variable pigmentation and central pinkish area, was confirmed histologically to be a basal cell papilloma.

Management

If you think that the lesion might be a malignant melanoma, refer the patient for a specialist opinion. Curettage and cautery is inappropriate treatment for a melanoma. Ellipse excision may be necessary to confirm the diagnosis but, as this is an inappropriate procedure for a basal cell papilloma, the decision to do this is best taken by a specialist.

INTRADERMAL MELANOCYTIC NAEVUS VERSUS BASAL CELL CARCINOMA

Basal cell carcinomas and benign intradermal melanocytic naevi are both commonest on the face and both can have the typical nodular cystic appearance of basal cell carcinoma, with overlying telangiectasia (Figure 2.2).

Management

The best treatment for a benign melanocytic intradermal naevus is shave excision, whereas a basal cell carcinoma should be treated by ellipse excision. If

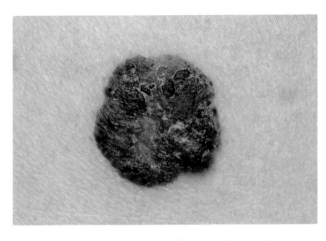

Figure 2.1 Variable pigmentation and irregular outline suggest the diagnosis of malignant melanoma. This was in fact a basal cell papilloma.

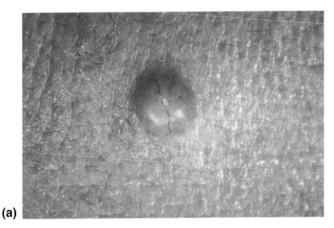

(a)

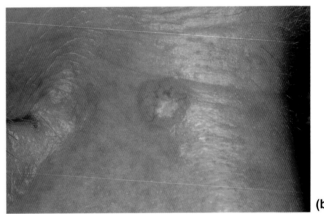

(b)

Figure 2.2 **(a)** Despite this lesion having a cystic nodular appearance with telangiectasia, it was shown histologically to be a benign intradermal melanocytic naevus rather than a nodular basal cell carcinoma.
(b) This lesion looks very similar to **(a)**, but was shown histologically to be a nodular basal cell carcinoma.

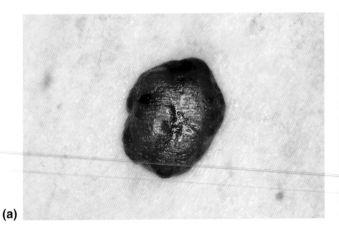

(a)

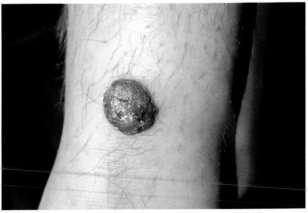

(b)

Figure 2.3 **(a)** This rapidly enlarging lesion was confirmed as a pyogenic granuloma, although it shows some similarities with **(b)**. **(b)** This rapidly enlarging lesion bled when caught, but was found to be a nodular malignant melanoma. There is some pigment present, although much of the tumour is amelanotic.

you have doubt about the diagnosis refer for a specialist opinion.

PYOGENIC GRANULOMA VERSUS AMELANOTIC MALIGNANT MELANOMA

Although pyogenic granuloma is much commoner than amelanotic malignant melanoma, the two conditions can look similar (Figure 2.3).

Both enlarge rapidly and develop into a juicy nodular lesion. Pyogenic granuloma is usually more vascular and bleeds more readily. Although pigment is absent from an amelanotic melanoma by definition, a small amount is sometimes visible using a magnifying lens. Sometimes the patient will describe a small pre-existing pigmented lesion.

Management

Even though the lesion is almost certain to be a pyogenic granuloma, it should be removed urgently (within 1–2 weeks) and the specimen sent, as always, for histological examination. Curettage and cautery is the appropriate procedure because the diagnosis of pyogenic granuloma is the most likely. If the lesion is subsequently shown to be an amelanotic malignant melanoma, further surgery can be arranged.

SUBUNGUAL HAEMATOMA VERSUS SUBUNGUAL MALIGNANT MELANOMA

A brown tumour beneath the nail will often be mistaken for a subungual haematoma (Figure 2.4(a)).

In the absence of a history of trauma to the nail the diagnosis of subungual haematoma can be very difficult to make. A longitudinal pigmented band in the nail suggests melanocytic proliferation. With time a subungual malignant melanoma will lead to longitudinal splitting of the nail, oozing, paronychia, nail dystrophy and finally destruction of the nail (Figure 2.4(b)). The prognosis of subungual malignant melanoma is poor and it is an important condition to diagnose early. It is therefore unacceptable to wait and see whether the nail grows out normally, as always happens when a subungual haematoma resolves. Most specialists have a very low threshold for performing a nail biopsy if there is any possibility that a subungual lesion is melanocytic.

Management

Refer the patient urgently to a specialist (to be seen within 1–2 weeks), with a view to an urgent nail biopsy.

SOLAR KERATOSIS VERSUS BOWEN'S DISEASE VERSUS SQUAMOUS CELL CARCINOMA

In patients with many solar keratoses it is tempting to treat multiple lesions with cryotherapy. Although treating a patch of Bowen's disease with liquid nitrogen will cause no adverse effects, cryotherapy is the wrong treatment for squamous cell carcinoma. Before treating it, look carefully at any presumed solar keratosis for evidence of induration and infiltration of the surrounding skin and question the patient about recent change in the lesion (Figure 2.5).

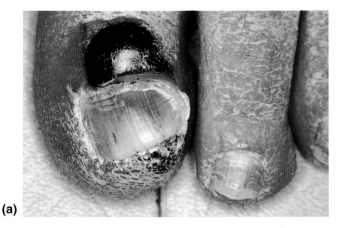

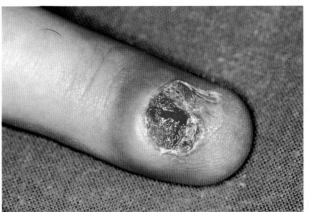

(a)   **(b)**

Figure 2.4 **(a)** Subungual haematoma. **(b)** Subungual malignant melanoma, which has destroyed the nail.

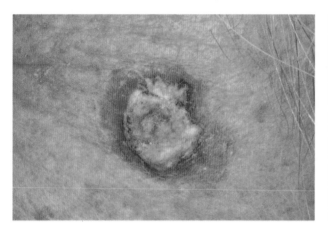

Figure 2.5 This keratotic lesion has an inflamed indurated base. The crust was lifted and a biopsy was taken. Histopathology showed evidence of full-thickness epidermal dysplasia with microinvasion consistent with a very early squamous cell carcinoma.

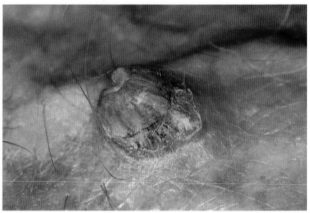

Figure 2.6 Typical example of a cutaneous horn. This is a clinical, not a pathological diagnosis.

Lifting the crust may reveal a nodule or an ulcer if the lesion is an SCC.

Management

If you have any doubt about the diagnosis you should refer the patient for a specialist opinion.

CUTANEOUS HORN

A cutaneous horn represents an abnormal proliferation of keratin. It is a clinical and not a pathological diagnosis (Figure 2.6).

There are several possible underlying pathological processes that lead to the development of such a lesion. A viral wart is the most likely cause in a young patient, whereas a solar keratosis is most probable on light-exposed skin in an older patient. Squamous cell carcinoma is the most important differential diagnosis and should always be borne in mind.

Management

It is most important to establish a histological diagnosis by examining the tissue at the base of the horn. Examination of the keratin alone is of no value. Curettage and cautery or ellipse excision will provide the necessary information.

Chapter 3

Management: the histology report

PRINCIPLES

Should you send a specimen for histological examination even if you are absolutely certain what it is?

The only safe answer is **yes, always.**

This is for two reasons.

- No matter how certain you are of the clinical diagnosis, you may be wrong. All pathologists occasionally come across epidermoid cysts containing tumours, or seemingly benign lesions that turn out to be something rare and sinister.
- The patient from whom you have removed some simple benign lesion may subsequently develop a completely unconnected malignancy, often years later. Unless you have firm evidence that what you removed was benign you may be unable to defend yourself against the charge that the original lesion was malignant and that you were negligent in missing the diagnosis.

The only safe policy is to submit everything you remove to the histology laboratory.

PATHOLOGY SPECIMENS

Throughout this book we make the point that you should not remove a lesion without first making a clinical diagnosis. On the basis of that diagnosis you will decide what procedure is most appropriate. You should provide the histopathologist with as much relevant clinical information as possible and send the specimen properly fixed, identified and orientated.

It is very helpful to put in a marker suture on one side of the specimen, with a simple drawing on the request form showing the specimen's orientation. Remember also to record any previous cryosurgery since this may alter the histological appearance of the specimen. Although curettings are disrupted tissue they too should be sent since they can provide satisfactory diagnostic information.

Be very careful if you remove multiple lesions from the same patient. If you put a number of specimens in the same pot and one turns out to be malignant you will be unable to identify the culprit. Always send specimens in separate numbered pots, preferably with a diagram illustrating the source of each one.

It is important not only to send all specimens to the laboratory but also to record in the notes that you have done so. Finally, it is vital to have a system for tracking each specimen and for making sure that every result has been received, checked and, most importantly, understood (Chapter 5).

INTERPRETING THE HISTOLOGY REPORT

Usually the histology report will be self-explanatory. Sometimes, however, it may be more difficult to interpret. It may be couched in unfamiliar technical terms or you may be unsure of the clinical implications for managing your patient. The rest of this chapter is based on real examples and discusses what action to take in each case.

PIGMENTED LESIONS

Pigmented lesions form the largest group of lesions excised in general practice. The vast majority will be either benign melanocytic naevi (moles) or basal cell papillomas (seborrhoeic keratoses). More rarely, a malignant melanoma is removed inadvertently.

Benign melanocytic naevi

The report will typically read:
- 'dermal melanocytic naevus, completely excised'
- 'compound melanocytic naevus, completely removed'
- 'junctional melanocytic naevus, completely excised'.

These histological descriptions correspond to the clinical descriptions elsewhere in the book. The distinction between compound, junctional and intra-dermal is of no consequence with regard to managing the patient. Although the term 'benign' is often not included in the descriptive report of a melanocytic naevus, the examples above are all benign. Consequently, reports suggesting incomplete excision should cause no concern.

Dysplastic melanocytic naevi

To many clinicians the term 'dysplasia' suggests premalignant change. It is therefore very important to understand the use of the term in the context of the pigmented skin lesion. It is important to know firstly the amount of dysplasia (i.e. mild, moderate or severe), and secondly whether the lesion was solitary or one of many other melanocytic lesions. The simple guidelines below will ensure safe practice.

'JUNCTIONAL/COMPOUND MELANOCYTIC LESION WITH MILD DYSPLASIA'

- Whether completely or incompletely removed this report should cause no alarm for you or the patient.
- Many solitary benign naevi show mild dysplasia.
- If the patient has many other moles, in particular, odd-looking ones, then you may wish to seek reassurance from a dermatologist that the patient does not have the atypical mole syndrome (p. 10). This is associated with an increased incidence of malignant melanoma. Referral for a routine appointment is appropriate. While awaiting the hospital appointment the patient should be advised to report if any other pigmented lesion changes in size, shape or colour.

'JUNCTIONAL/COMPOUND MELANOCYTIC NAEVUS WITH MODERATE DYSPLASIA'

This report should not be ignored or inadvertently filed before careful assessment and appropriate action. Management depends on whether or not the lesion is completely excised and whether or not the patient has multiple moles.
- The patient should be reassured that, although the mole was active, it was not malignant.
- Because the diagnosis of malignant melanoma has implications for patients obtaining life insurance, it is important to stress to the patient that the diagnosis is not malignant melanoma.

Complete excision, very few other moles and no atypical moles
- No further surgery is necessary provided the lesion is reported as completely removed.
- Advise the patient to return for review if new pigmentation develops within the scar.
- A recurrence at any time demands urgent referral to the dermatology department, where the initial histology can be reviewed and appropriate management instituted.

Complete excision, multiple moles and/or several atypical-looking moles
- If the other moles look benign, refer for a routine dermatological opinion to consider the possibility of atypical mole syndrome.
- If any of the other moles look worrying, refer for an urgent dermatological opinion.
- Give simple advice about checking moles for change in size, shape and colour. Expedite out-patient appointment if any other moles change and cause concern. Make the patient aware of the harmful effects of sun exposure and give advice about sunscreens and sun avoidance.

Incomplete excision, very few other moles and no other worrying or unusual moles
- Take advice, preferably from your dermatologist, by telephone. The dermatologist will probably arrange to review the specimen with the histopathologist and then discuss management with you.
- If this is not practicable, refer urgently for excision of scar.

- If you feel confident, arrange to excise the scar yourself. Meanwhile either discuss the histology report with the dermatologist or refer the patient for a routine dermatology out-patient appointment.

Incomplete excision, multiple moles and/or several other unusual moles

The guidelines above apply, but in addition:
- ensure that the patient has a dermatological opinion in weeks rather than months;
- give simple advice about checking moles for change in size, shape and colour. Expedite out-patient appointment if any other moles change and cause concern. Make patient 'sun aware'.

'MELANOCYTIC NAEVUS WITH SEVERE DYSPLASIA'

This is much more worrying, as the interpretation of severely dysplastic changes varies. Some histopathologists consider severe dysplasia to indicate melanoma *in situ*. In such cases the histology should be reviewed by the dermatologist and histopathologist together to plan future management.

Severe dysplasia, complete excision

Although the time scale is not vital, request an urgent out-patient appointment for everyone's peace of mind. Include the histology reference number in your letter so that the histology can be reviewed before the patient attends. If there is a high level of anxiety then telephone the dermatology department and ask for the histology to be reviewed at an early stage.

Severe dysplasia, incomplete excision

We would suggest urgent referral. Arrange an early out-patient appointment (within 1–2 weeks) by telephone.

Malignant melanoma

Most pigmented lesions removed in general practice are benign. Most malignant melanomas are excised in hospital. Occasionally, however, a report will appear on your desk as follows: 'Skin with a superficial spreading malignant melanoma. The tumour depth is 0.9 mm. The mitotic rate is high and there is a marked lymphocytic reaction. Surface margin is 2.3 mm; deep margin 3.5 mm.'

This is a real 'heart sink' report which usually comes as a complete surprise, and often you cannot even put a face to the name on the report. How should you react?

Firstly do not panic, but read the report carefully and ask two questions.
- **What is the thickness of the tumour?** The single most important factor in prognosis of malignant melanoma is the tumour thickness at presentation (p. 28). Thin tumours (less than 1 mm) have a very good prognosis, thick tumours (greater than 3 mm) have a very poor prognosis. Figures for 5-year survival are given in Chapter 1 (p. 28).
- **Is the tumour completely removed** and, if so, by what excision margin?

With the answers to these two important questions you can decide how to proceed. But remember, even if the excision is incomplete you have not worsened the prognosis, provided you act promptly.

MALIGNANT MELANOMA, BRESLOW THICKNESS LESS THAN 1 MM, COMPLETELY EXCISED WITH 2 MM EXCISION MARGIN

- This patient has an excellent outlook, with a 5-year survival figure of 98%.
- Further surgery is necessary to give a 1 cm margin of excision.
- Arrange an urgent dermatology out-patient appointment (1–2 weeks). Arrange to review the patient within the next few days and give this appointment to the patient yourself at the consultation. Make sure the dermatologist receives a copy of the histology report before the patient is seen at out-patients.
- When you review the patient explain the diagnosis in a very positive way. Many people still associate malignant melanoma with a very poor prognosis and it is important to reassure the patient that early surgical excision leads to complete cure. Discuss the need and reasons for further surgery.

MALIGNANT MELANOMA, BRESLOW THICKNESS GREATER THAN 1 MM, COMPLETELY OR INCOMPLETELY EXCISED

In this group of patients the outcome is likely to be worse. The prognosis and management will depend on the age of the patient, the site of the lesion, the type of melanoma and whether there is any evidence of metastatic disease. Previously, wide surgical excision, with or without lymph node dissection, was the treatment of choice in this group of patients. There is now good evidence that extensive surgery does little to influence the outcome. The recommended excision margin for melanomas up to 2 mm in thickness is 1 cm. The necessary margin for thicker tumours is still debated. A reasonable management strategy is as follows.

- Arrange an urgent out-patient assessment (1–2 weeks) by a plastic surgeon. Make sure the referral contains a copy of the histology report.
- Discuss the diagnosis with your patient in general terms. Try to be positive but explain that your knowledge of the outlook is limited. Advise the patient of the referral you have arranged and warn that further surgery may be necessary.
- Malignant melanoma is neither radiosensitive nor responsive to chemotherapy, so referral to a radiotherapist or oncologist at this stage is inappropriate.

SOLAR (ACTINIC) KERATOSIS

Usually you will elect not to excise these lesions. However if you do remove them by curettage, the curettings should be sent for histopathological assessment. This will usually confirm your clinical diagnosis and no further action will be required. It is reasonable to tell the patient that the lesion removed was a 'sun spot' and to take the opportunity of discussing the dangers of excessive sun exposure. The tendency for solar keratoses to be more active in the summer and less active in the winter is worth mentioning.

'SOLAR KERATOSIS WITH MILD/MODERATE DYSPLASIA'

All solar keratoses show some degree of dysplasia, from mild through to severe. Provided the dysplastic change is confined to the epidermis there is no cause for concern.

IF THE WORD 'MICROINVASION' APPEARS IN THE REPORT

This may indicate an early squamous cell carcinoma. Squamous cell carcinoma arising in a solar keratosis is usually very slowly growing.

- Refer the patient for a dermatological opinion within about 2–4 weeks. The histology will be reviewed and further surgery arranged as appropriate.

- The patient can be reassured but should be advised that the biopsy report has suggested the presence of very early skin cancer. Again it is important to explain that this is non-melanoma skin cancer and that there is a possibility that a further very minor surgical procedure may be required. Stress that the outlook is excellent and that spread is very unlikely.
- If there is no evidence of a residual lesion and the patient is elderly and frail, arrange to review at 3, 6 and 12 months. Refer if there is any evidence of recurrence.

BOWEN'S DISEASE

This is sometimes reported as intra-epithelial or intra-epidermal dysplasia, i.e. dysplasia extending throughout the epidermis. If left it will inevitably progress to squamous cell carcinoma although the period of latency may be many years.

'PATCH OF BOWEN'S DISEASE, COMPLETELY EXCISED'

- Review the patient and check that this was a solitary patch, that the scar has healed and that there is no clinical evidence of residual tumour. If so, arrange follow-up at 3, 6 and 12 months. Refer if the lesion recurs.
- Check the patient for other non-melanoma skin cancers.
- Reassure the patient that the lesion was harmless but that if it had been left it would have progressed to a skin cancer many years later.
- Advise the patient to return early if the lesion recurs or if any other persistent or non-healing lesions develop.
- If on review you find other skin tumours you should arrange dermatological assessment relatively urgently (about 4–6 weeks). Next week if you discover a melanoma!
- If the patient's skin is generally sun damaged, you may prefer to refer the patient to the dermatology out-patients for a general skin examination.

'PATCH OF BOWEN'S DISEASE, INCOMPLETELY EXCISED'

- This can be managed in a number of different ways depending on such factors as site, size of residual lesion and age of patient.
- Refer for dermatological assessment within about 4–6 weeks.

KERATOACANTHOMA

A report of such a lesion will nearly always conclude: 'Although the clinical history and histological appearances support the diagnosis of keratoacanthoma, the diagnosis of squamous cell carcinoma cannot be completely excluded on this specimen.'

This report must not be filed and forgotten! Consider carefully how to proceed. Much will depend on your preoperative clinical diagnosis, the site of the lesion, the age of the patient and whether or not excision is complete. If the clinical diagnosis of keratoacanthoma is in any doubt the lesion should be managed as a squamous cell carcinoma.

'KERATOACANTHOMA, COMPLETELY EXCISED'
- No further surgery is necessary.
- Tell the patient that this was almost certainly a benign lesion but that occasionally it can recur. Advise the patient to attend for regular review but to return earlier if the lesion recurs.
- Arrange regular review at 3, 6 and 12 months and refer if there is any evidence of recurrence. If the lesion recurs this suggests that the original lesion was a squamous cell carcinoma. The patient should be referred urgently (appointment within 2 weeks). This type of squamous cell carcinoma is more aggressive than that arising in a solar keratosis.

'KERATOACANTHOMA, INCOMPLETELY EXCISED'
- Because of the risk of missing and treating inappropriately a squamous cell carcinoma you may prefer to discuss the patient with your dermatologist. Alternatively an urgent hospital referral may be appropriate, requesting the patient to be seen within about 3 weeks.
- Usually further surgery or radiotherapy is indicated to remove any residual lesion. Occasionally no further treatment is necessary and a wait-and-see approach can be adopted. This decision is best taken by a specialist.
- Reassure the patient that the lesion was almost certainly benign but that it was not completely removed and that it may rarely recur. Advise the patient that this lesion can sometimes turn out to be a type of skin cancer, again stressing the point that this is a good type of cancer to have and is nothing to do with mole skin cancer. Even if it subsequently becomes clear that it was a skin cancer, the outlook is good.

SQUAMOUS CELL CARCINOMA

The realization that you have removed a squamous cell carcinoma usually comes as an alarming surprise. You should consider the management in two stages. First, management of the lesion itself. Secondly, the rest of the skin should be checked for other non-melanoma skin cancers which are known to develop and will need treating.

'SQUAMOUS CELL CARCINOMA, COMPLETELY EXCISED'
- Relax. If the patient is elderly or frail no further treatment is necessary. The patient should be reviewed at 3-, 6- and 12-month intervals. Refer the patient if the lesion recurs. Ideally, check the rest of the patient's skin.
- In younger patients, with or without obvious sun damage, consider referral for full skin check and education about non-melanoma skin cancer and sun avoidance. Referral is also an opportunity to review the histopathology and check the excision margins. Patients should be seen preferably within about 6–8 weeks of excision.
- Reassure the patient that the tumour has been completely removed. Explain that this is non-melanoma skin cancer, which may invade locally but doesn't usually spread internally. Further surgery is seldom necessary. Warn the patient that other non-melanoma skin cancers may occur and ask the patient to return if any other persistent or non-healing lesions develop.

'SQUAMOUS CELL CARCINOMA, INCOMPLETELY EXCISED'
- This is not such good news but there is still no need to panic. Refer the patient urgently as he/she will require further specialist assessment and treatment.
- Both plastic surgery and radiotherapy are used and you may refer directly to either of these departments. Alternatively you may wish to discuss the case with the dermatologist first.
- Occasionally a further small surgical procedure carried out by the dermatologist may suffice.
- Again be positive in your consultation with the patient, discussing the issues raised in the previous example. You should also discuss the need for referral and further treatment.

BASAL CELL CARCINOMA

Basal cell carcinomas (BCC) are very slow-growing, locally invasive tumours. Some GPs elect to excise them in the elderly and frail as this is more convenient for the patient. BCCs are sometimes discovered only after histopathological examination of an excised lesion. It is important to remember that, if a patient presents with one BCC, there is a one in five chance of a second tumour developing within the next 5 years. Follow-up involves looking both for recurrence and for second tumours. The patient is also more likely to have other non-melanoma skin cancers and solar keratoses.

Where possible, surgical excision is the preferred option for BCCs although radiotherapy is sometimes indicated. If you remove a BCC from a patient younger than 50 years old, particularly if there is more than one, it is worth referring the patient for a dermatological opinion to exclude the diagnosis of Gorlin's syndrome (a family cancer syndrome).

'NODULAR BASAL CELL CARCINOMA, COMPLETELY EXCISED'

- No further surgery is required.
- Reassure the patient that although this is skin cancer, it is the 'good' type of skin cancer that never spreads to any other part of the body and is not life-threatening. It is usually only a nuisance, but if left would continue to enlarge and invade locally.
- It is often useful to clarify that this is not 'mole' skin cancer. Many patients who have had a BCC removed will tell you at a later date that it was a melanoma.
- Review the patient at 3 and 6 months to look for recurrence and to ask about other non-healing lesions.
- Either ask the patient to return if the scar changes or arrange annual review if you feel the patient is unlikely to report with a recurrence or new tumour.

'NODULAR BASAL CELL CARCINOMA, INCOMPLETELY EXCISED'

- Further surgery is indicated, but only to remove residual tumour.
- There is no urgency about referral, but 4–6 weeks is preferable.
- Depending upon the site, arrange referral either to a dermatologist or a plastic surgeon.

- Discuss the diagnosis and prognosis as outlined above.

'MORPHOEIC BASAL CELL CARCINOMA ...' OR 'FEATURES OF A MORPHOEIC TYPE TUMOUR ARE SEEN'

- This is a rarer type of BCC which is more difficult to manage, and recurrence is more likely.
- Margins of excision are often difficult to define clinically and histologically.
- Refer to a radiotherapist, plastic surgeon or dermatologist for further assessment (within 4–6 weeks).
- Give positive advice to the patient about the diagnosis, as previously described, but warn about the need for further surgery or radiotherapy to prevent local recurrence.

'MULTICENTRIC BASAL CELL CARCINOMA ... THE MARGIN OF EXCISION IS LESS THAN THE DISTANCE BETWEEN TUMOUR NESTS'

- As the name implies these are 'many-centred' and are often more extensive than is first apparent. They are more likely to occur on the trunk and are frequently multiple (p. 25).
- Where the margin of excision is less than the distance between tumour nests you cannot be sure that the tumour is completely removed.
- In these tumours, even if the histology report indicates complete excision, the possibility remains of further residual tumour nests just outside the excision margin.
- Refer the patient to a dermatologist, to be seen within 6–8 weeks.
- If the lesion is clinically completely removed and the patient is elderly or frail, arrange review at 3 and 6 months. Annual review is only necessary if you think the patient would not report a recurrence.
- Once again the patient can be reassured that there is no cause for concern and that this type of skin cancer grows slowly and is only locally invasive. Wherever possible the patient should be instructed to check for recurrence and for other similar lesions, and to seek medical advice if worried about either.
- Hospital referral is indicated if a recurrence develops.

OTHER UNUSUAL REPORTS

If a fleshy lesion proves to be a neurofibroma or a Schwannoma you should establish whether the lesion was solitary. Check the whole of the patient's skin, looking for café-au-lait patches and axillary freckling. If you discover features of neurofibromatosis refer the patient for a full assessment. Remember, however, that a solitary neurofibroma may occur without the patient having neurofibromatosis. Eccrine hydradenomas and syringomas are relatively rare benign sweat gland tumours that are sometimes removed without a preoperative diagnosis.

THE BOTTOM LINE

- If you remove lesions only where you are confident of the clinical diagnosis, the histological diagnosis will rarely cause any difficulty.

- If you do not understand the report, do not ignore it. Ask your dermatologist or histopathologist for help.
- If you receive an unusual or unexpected report you should always evaluate it and decide on a management plan before discussing it with the patient.
- In the case of a surprising report, e.g. Kaposi's sarcoma in a teenager with no predisposing factors for HIV infection, the histology should be reviewed before discussing the diagnosis with the patient. If the lesion proves to be benign you will have saved the patient a period of unnecessary anxiety.
- Seek specialist advice if the histology report is particularly unusual or unexpected, e.g. a basal cell carcinoma in a 25-year-old or a keratoacanthoma in a 30-year-old. The skin lesion could be a marker of a family cancer syndrome requiring screening for internal malignancy.

Chapter 4
Gallery

FRECKLES

SYNONYM Ephelides

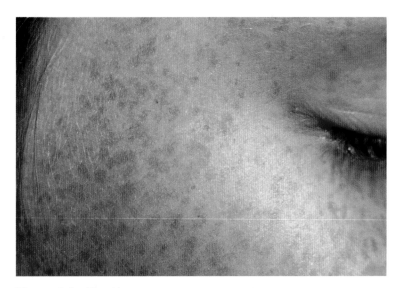

Figure 4.1 Freckles.

FEATURES (p. 6)

Benign

Incidence

Common

Site

Any part of the body; commonest on sun-exposed skin

Clinical features (Figure 4.1)

- Pigmented macules
- Diameter 1–3 mm
- Darker after sun exposure
- Usually family history

ACCEPTABLE MANAGEMENT

Leave alone

RECOMMENDED TREATMENT

Leave alone

TREATMENT TO AVOID

Excision

CAUTIONARY NOTES

Axillary freckling and/or café-au-lait patches are/is a marker of neurofibromatosis

LENTIGO

SYNONYM None

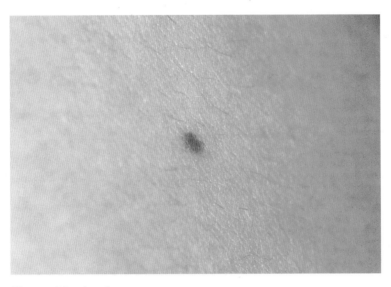

Figure 4.2 Lentigo.

FEATURES (p. 6)

Benign

Incidence

Common

Site

Any part of the body; commonest on sun-exposed skin

Clinical features (Figure 4.2)

- Pigmented macule
- Diameter 1–3 mm
- Often solitary
- Commonly multiple in sun-damaged skin (solar lentigo)

ACCEPTABLE MANAGEMENT

Leave alone

RECOMMENDED TREATMENT

Leave alone

TREATMENT TO AVOID

Excision

CAUTIONARY NOTES

Brown patch of lentigo on face may be Hutchinson's freckle

BENIGN MELANOCYTIC NAEVUS: JUNCTIONAL MELANOCYTIC NAEVUS

SYNONYM Mole, melanoma

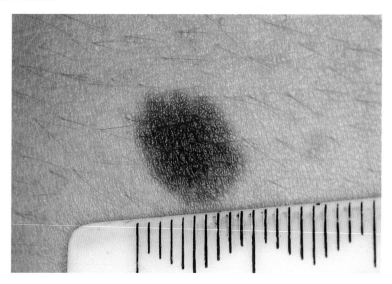

Figure 4.3   Junctional melanocytic naevus.

FEATURES (p. 7)

Benign

Incidence
- Common
- Commoner in fair-skinned people

Site
Occurs on any part of the body

Clinical features (Figure 4.3)
- Sometimes variably pigmented
- Usually less than 1 cm diameter
- Commonest in puberty and early adult life, absent in elderly
- May evolve into compound or intradermal melanocytic naevus (p. 8–9)

ACCEPTABLE MANAGEMENT
- Leave alone if confident of diagnosis
- Refer if uncertain of diagnosis
- Consider cosmetic excision with 2 mm margin if patient requests it

RECOMMENDED TREATMENT
- Leave alone if confident of diagnosis
- Ellipse excision (p. 111) with 2 mm margin if patient requests it

TREATMENT TO AVOID
- Cryotherapy contraindicated
- Avoid sites where cosmetic result may be unsatisfactory

CAUTIONARY NOTES
Differential diagnosis is malignant melanoma

BENIGN MELANOCYTIC NAEVUS: COMPOUND MELANOCYTIC NAEVUS

SYNONYM Mole, melanoma

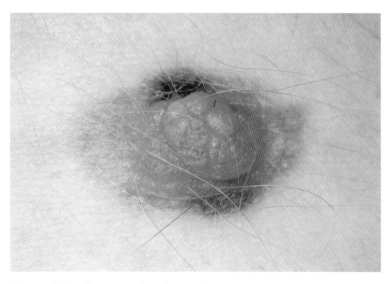

Figure 4.4　Compound melanocytic naevus.

FEATURES (p. 8–9)

Benign

Incidence

Common

Site

Any site, but commoner on the face and trunk

Clinical features (Figure 4.4)

- Raised pigmented lesion, not crusted
- Usually less than 1 cm diameter
- Sometimes hairy
- May be multiple
- Typically appears in puberty, absent in elderly
- May evolve to intradermal naevus (p. 8–9)

ACCEPTABLE MANAGEMENT

- Leave alone if confident of diagnosis
- Refer if diagnostic uncertainty
- Consider cosmetic removal if patient requests it
- Shave excision preferable
- Ellipse excision only if linear scar acceptable

RECOMMENDED TREATMENT

- Leave alone
- Shave excision (p. 119)

TREATMENT TO AVOID

- Curettage and cautery
- Cryotherapy
- Avoid sites where cosmetic result may be unsatisfactory

CAUTIONARY NOTES

- Discuss likely cosmetic result
- Warn about pigmentation recurring and hairs regrowing in scar of shave excision

BENIGN MELANOCYTIC NAEVUS: INTRADERMAL MELANOCYTIC NAEVUS

SYNONYM Mole

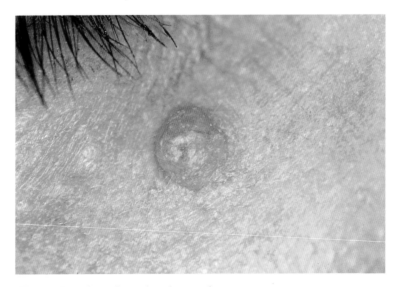

Figure 4.5 Intradermal melanocytic naevus.

FEATURES (p. 9)

Benign

Incidence

Common

Site

Any site but most commonly seen on the face

Clinical features (Figure 4.5)

- Raised, non-pigmented
- May be hairy
- Usually less than 1 cm diameter
- May be multiple
- Occurs in adults but not in elderly

ACCEPTABLE MANAGEMENT

- Leave alone if confident of diagnosis
- Refer if diagnostic uncertainty
- Shave excision

RECOMMENDED TREATMENT

- Leave alone
- Shave excision (p. 119)

TREATMENT TO AVOID

- Cryotherapy
- Ellipse excision
- Curettage and cautery
- Sites where the cosmetic result may be unsatisfactory

CAUTIONARY NOTES

- Differential diagnosis from basal cell carcinoma sometimes difficult
- Warn about hairs regrowing in scar of shave excision

BENIGN MELANOCYTIC NAEVUS: HALO NAEVUS

SYNONYM Sutton's halo naevus

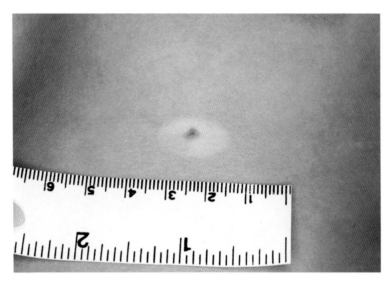

Figure 4.6 Halo naevus.

FEATURES (p. 9)

Benign

Incidence

Less common than other types of benign pigmented naevus

Site

Commonest on the trunk

Clinical features (Figure 4.6)

- Commonest in adolescents and young adults
- Flat pigmented melanocytic naevus (usually junctional) becomes surrounded by an area of hypopigmentation
- Central melanocytic naevus becomes smaller and eventually disappears
- Area of hypopigmentation, in general, repigments eventually

ACCEPTABLE MANAGEMENT

- Leave alone if confident of diagnosis
- Review patient at intervals to check that the lesion is behaving as expected
- Refer if the central pigmented lesion enlarges or looks worrying

RECOMMENDED TREATMENT

- Leave alone
- Refer for reassurance if necessary

TREATMENT TO AVOID

- Cryotherapy
- Excision

CAUTIONARY NOTES

Refer if atypical presentation

MELANOCYTIC NAEVUS: ATYPICAL MELANOCYTIC NAEVUS

SYNONYM Dysplastic naevus (avoid this term)

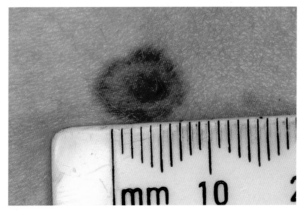 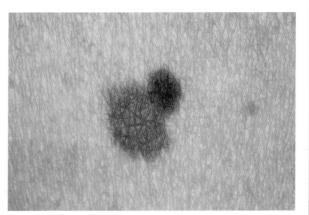

Figure 4.7(a) and (b)   Atypical melanocytic naevus.

FEATURES (p. 10)

Benign

Incidence

- Less common than other melanocytic naevi
- 5% of the population will have one

Site

Commoner on trunk

Clinical features (Figure 4.7)

- Large (greater than 5 mm) pigmented lesion
- Irregular border
- May be variably pigmented, sometimes with pinkish inflamed appearance

ACCEPTABLE MANAGEMENT

- Leave alone if lesion unchanging and confident of diagnosis
- Refer for diagnostic confirmation
- Check patient for features of atypical mole syndrome (p. 10)
- Consider ellipse excision with 2 mm margin if patient requests removal

RECOMMENDED TREATMENT

- Leave alone if confident of diagnosis
- Refer for diagnostic confirmation

TREATMENT TO AVOID

- Cryotherapy
- Shave excision
- Curettage and cautery contraindicated

CAUTIONARY NOTES

Beware: differential diagnosis is malignant melanoma

CONGENITAL MELANOCYTIC NAEVUS

SYNONYM None

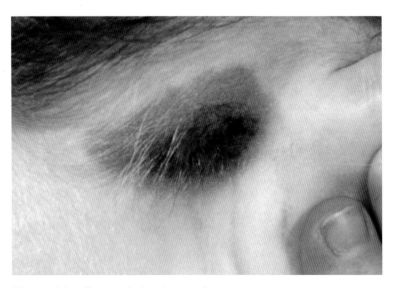

Figure 4.8 Congenital melanocytic naevus.

FEATURES (p. 11)

Benign, although increased risk of malignant change

Incidence

Solitary small ones not uncommon; large 'garment' or 'bathing trunk' naevi rare

Site

- Solitary small lesions can occur at any site
- Larger lesions usually on trunk or can involve a whole limb

Clinical features (Figure 4.8)

- By definition present at birth or in the first few weeks of life
- Size variable
- Dark brown and often raised
- Often has mamillary projections
- May be hairy, sometimes very hairy

ACCEPTABLE MANAGEMENT

- Refer patients with large lesions to plastic surgeon or dermatologist
- Advise patient to check naevus regularly for any changes
- If a congenital naevus changes in size, shape or colour, refer
- Management of small lesions debatable – some dermatologists believe that congenital naevi should be excised wherever possible because of risk of malignant change; consider referral to dermatologist to discuss the latest view

RECOMMENDED TREATMENT

Refer

TREATMENT TO AVOID

Cryotherapy

CAUTIONARY NOTES

Probable increased risk of malignant change: take seriously any history of change in a congenital naevus

BENIGN MELANOCYTIC NAEVUS: BLUE NAEVUS

SYNONYM None

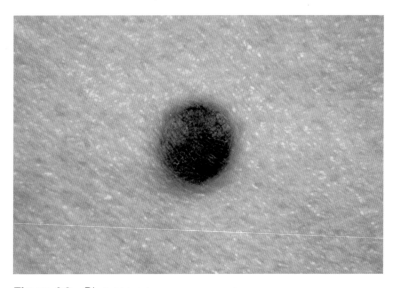

Figure 4.9   Blue naevus.

FEATURES (p. 11)

Benign

Incidence

Less common than other melanocytic naevi

Site

Commoner on the extremities

Clinical features (Figure 4.9)

- Appears in childhood or early adult life
- Usually solitary
- Distinctive dark blue/slate grey colour
- Slightly raised
- Diameter more than 1 cm

ACCEPTABLE MANAGEMENT

- Leave alone if confident of clinical diagnosis
- Refer if diagnostic uncertainty or lesion changing
- Consider ellipse excision (p. 111) with 2 mm margin if patient requests it

RECOMMENDED TREATMENT

- Leave alone if confident of diagnosis, refer if not
- For cosmetic excisions remove by ellipse excision with 2 mm margin (p. 111)

TREATMENT TO AVOID

- Cryotherapy
- Curettage and cautery
- Avoid sites where cosmetic result may be unsatisfactory

CAUTIONARY NOTES

May be difficult to distinguish from malignant melanoma

MELANOCYTIC NAEVUS: SPITZ NAEVUS

SYNONYM Juvenile melanoma

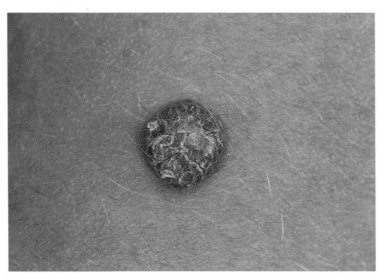

Figure 4.10 Spitz naevus.

FEATURES (p. 12)

Usually benign

Incidence

Rare

Site

Commonest on cheeks

Clinical features (Figure 4.10)

- Commonest in young children, can occur in adults
- Red or reddish-brown firm nodule
- Rapidly enlarging at first, then static
- May be up to 1–2 cm in diameter

ACCEPTABLE MANAGEMENT

Refer

RECOMMENDED TREATMENT

Refer

TREATMENT TO AVOID

Avoid managing the patient yourself

CAUTIONARY NOTES

The histology may resemble a malignant melanoma. This can be very worrying in the case of a small child. Refer for specialist management.

BASAL CELL PAPILLOMA

SYNONYM Seborrhoeic keratosis, seborrhoeic wart, senile keratosis, senile wart

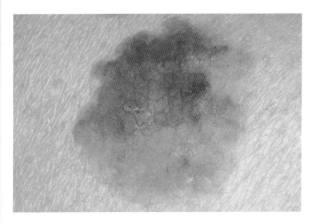 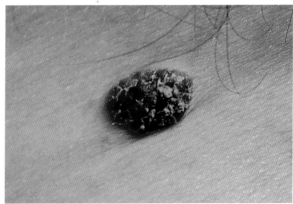

Figure 4.11(a) and (b)   Basal cell papilloma (seborrhoeic keratosis).

FEATURES (p. 12–14)

Benign

Incidence

Very common

Site

Commonest on trunk

Clinical features (Figure 4.11)

- Older patients
- Often multiple
- Crusted superficial lesions, greasy appearance
- New lesions develop over time
- No spontaneous resolution, crust may fall off

ACCEPTABLE MANAGEMENT

- Leave alone if certain of diagnosis
- Curettage and cautery
- Cryotherapy
- Refer if diagnostic doubt

RECOMMENDED TREATMENT

- Leave alone
- Curettage and cautery (p. 115–19)

TREATMENT TO AVOID

Ellipse excision is inappropriate

CAUTIONARY NOTES

Always send curettings for histological examination

SKIN TAGS

SYNONYM Warts, papillomas, fibro-epithelial polyps

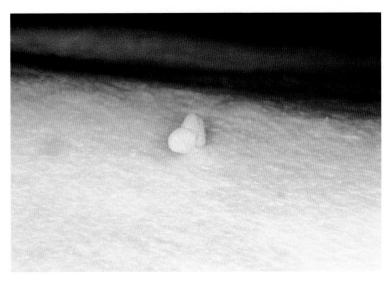

Figure 4.12 Skin tags.

FEATURES (p. 14)

Benign

Incidence

Common

Site

Commonest in axillae, groins and neck

Clinical features (Figure 4.12)

- Small (2–3 mm), fleshy pedunculated lesions
- Usually multiple
- Increase in number with age

ACCEPTABLE MANAGEMENT

- Snip excision
- Cautery

RECOMMENDED TREATMENT

- Snip excision (p. 120)
- Cautery (p. 118)
- Patients can snip off small ones themselves

TREATMENT TO AVOID

- Ellipse excision
- Tying cotton round the base; this produces nasty inflammatory response with scarring

CAUTIONARY NOTES

New tags often appear in predisposed individuals

EPIDERMOID CYST

SYNONYM Sebaceous cyst, pilar cyst, epithelial cyst

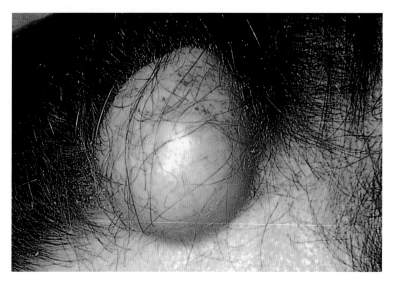

Figure 4.13 Epidermoid (pilar) cyst.

FEATURES (p. 14)

Benign

Incidence
- Common, particularly in young and middle-aged adults
- May occur as part of acne

Site

Common on head, neck, chest and back.

Clinical features (Figure 4.13)
- Cystic lesion usually 1–2 cm in diameter
- Overlying skin normal
- Keratin-filled punctum sometimes seen
- Contents have semisolid cheese appearance
- Cyst may become inflamed

ACCEPTABLE MANAGEMENT
- Leave alone if asymptomatic
- Excise if cosmetic nuisance
- If enlarged and inflamed consider incision and drainage, followed later by elective excision
- If part of acne vulgaris, treat acne first; acne cysts often difficult to remove

RECOMMENDED TREATMENT

Excision unless acutely inflamed (p. 112–14)

TREATMENT TO AVOID
- Incision and drainage except when acutely inflamed
- Incision and drainage of acne cysts
- Excision of acne cysts unless acne is quiet

CAUTIONARY NOTES

Cysts that have been inflamed on more than one occasion may be technically difficult to remove

DERMATOFIBROMA
SYNONYM Histiocytoma

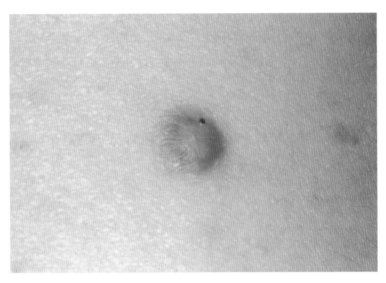

Figure 4.14　Dermatofibroma (histiocytoma).

FEATURES (p. 15)

Benign

Incidence

Common

Site

Commonest on lower leg

Clinical features (Figure 4.14)
- Particularly common in young women
- Firm itchy dermal nodule (0.5–1 cm diameter)
- Overlying skin usually normal colour but sometimes pigmented

ACCEPTABLE MANAGEMENT
- Leave alone if confident of diagnosis
- Ellipse excision (p. 111)

RECOMMENDED TREATMENT

Leave alone

TREATMENT TO AVOID

Avoid any treatment if confident of diagnosis

CAUTIONARY NOTES
- Always warn patient about scarring
- Resulting scar on the lower limb may look worse than dermatofibroma
- Healing on the lower limb is often poor

SPIDER NAEVUS
SYNONYM None

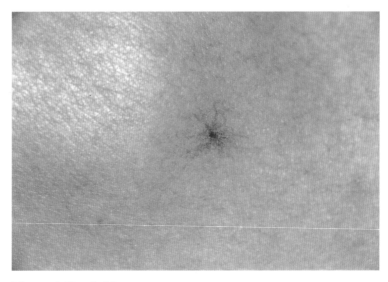

Figure 4.15   Spider naevus.

FEATURES (p. 16)

Incidence
Common, particularly in young women and especially during pregnancy

Site
Head, neck, arms and trunk

Clinical features (Figure 4.15)
- Small, red vascular lesions
- Usually solitary, sometimes multiple
- Blanch on pressure
- Often resolve spontaneously, particularly those occurring in pregnancy

ACCEPTABLE MANAGEMENT
- Leave alone
- Treat with cold point cautery (p. 118–19)
- Treat with Hyfrecator
- Refer to dermatologist for treatment with Hyfrecator or cold point cautery

RECOMMENDED TREATMENT
Leave alone

TREATMENT TO AVOID
- Excision
- Cryotherapy

CAUTIONARY NOTES
Solitary spider naevi are common; very large numbers of spider naevi occur in chronic liver disease

CAMPBELL DE MORGAN SPOT
SYNONYM Cherry angioma

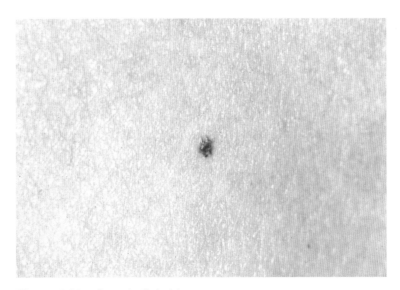

Figure 4.16   Campbell de Morgan spots.

FEATURES (p. 16)

Benign

Incidence

Very common, particularly in the middle-aged and elderly

Site

Usually on trunk

Clinical features (Figure 4.16)

- Small, cherry red spots, up to 5 mm in diameter
- Usually multiple
- Slightly raised
- Derived from blood vessels; histologically reported as angiokeratomas

ACCEPTABLE MANAGEMENT

Leave alone

RECOMMENDED TREATMENT

Leave alone

TREATMENT TO AVOID

Excision – lesions are usually multiple and new ones continue to develop

CAUTIONARY NOTES

Multiple angiokeratomas occur in young males in the rare but serious Anderson Fabry's disease (angiokeratoma corporis diffusum)

PYOGENIC GRANULOMA

SYNONYM Granuloma pyogenicum, granuloma telangiectaticum

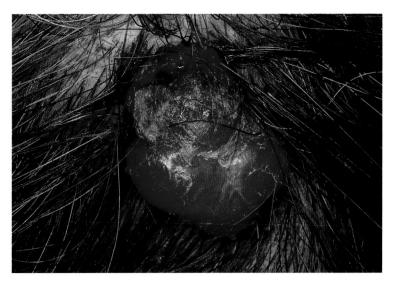

Figure 4.17 Pyogenic granuloma.

FEATURES (p. 16–17)

Benign

Incidence

Not very common

Site

Commonest on the extremities

Clinical features (Figure 4.17)

- Occur at any age but commonest in children and young adults
- Rapidly enlarging lesion
- Bright red, up to 10 mm diameter
- Bleeds profusely when touched

ACCEPTABLE MANAGEMENT

- Curettage and cautery, suture base if bleeds
- Ellipse excision

RECOMMENDED TREATMENT

Curettage and cautery (p. 115–19)

TREATMENT TO AVOID

Cryotherapy

CAUTIONARY NOTES

Differential diagnosis is amelanotic melanoma

VIRAL WARTS

TYPES Plantar wart (verruca), filiform wart, digital wart, plane wart

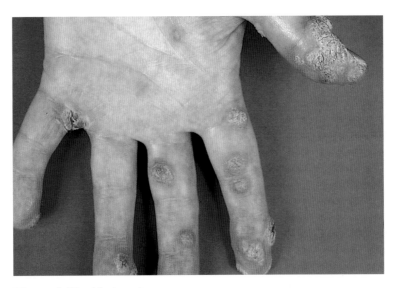

Figure 4.18 Viral warts.

FEATURES (p. 17–18)

Benign

Incidence

Common, particularly in childhood

Site

Commonest on hands and feet. Other sites include face

Clinical features (Figure 4.18)

- Hyperkeratosis consistent feature; amount varies depending upon site
- Plantar warts present as well-demarcated patch of hyperkeratosis of variable size (up to several centimetres) on the sole
- Digital and plantar warts display tiny black dots when pared down
- Filiform warts long and thin, often with narrow base
- Plane warts often extensive and resistant to treatment
- Most warts asymptomatic, cosmetic nuisance
- Usually resolve spontaneously without scarring, but may take years

ACCEPTABLE MANAGEMENT

- No treatment
- Keratolytic wart paints
- Formaldehyde soaks (3%) for plantar warts
- Liquid nitrogen cryotherapy (p. 120–23)

RECOMMENDED TREATMENT

Leave alone

TREATMENT TO AVOID

- Ellipse excision or curettage – wart often recurs in scar
- Cryotherapy in children

CAUTIONARY NOTES

- Many warts unresponsive to treatment
- Effective cryotherapy to plantar warts may leave patient unable to walk for several days after treatment; unjustifiable for asymptomatic lesion

MOLLUSCUM CONTAGIOSUM

SYNONYM None

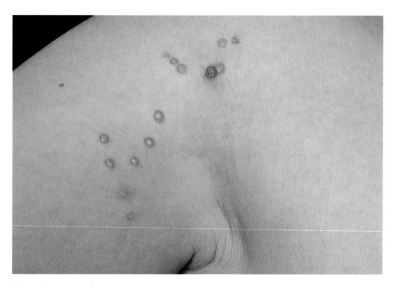

Figure 4.19 Molluscum contagiosum.

FEATURES (p. 17)

Benign

Incidence

Common, particularly in children

Site

Clusters, commonest on trunk and limbs; rare on face

Clinical features (Figure 4.19)

- Shiny, pearly white papules, usually umbilicated
- Diameter 5–10 mm
- Commonly multiple
- Often extensive in children with eczema; lesions spread by scratching
- Self-limiting within 6–9 months

ACCEPTABLE MANAGEMENT

- Leave alone
- Treat any atopic eczema to reduce likelihood of spread

RECOMMENDED TREATMENT

Leave alone

TREATMENT TO AVOID

Surgical excision

CAUTIONARY NOTES

Self-limiting, affects young children; avoid painful treatments

CHONDRODERMATITIS NODULARIS HELICIS

SYNONYM None

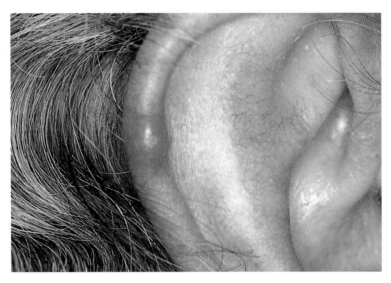

Figure 4.20 Chondrodermatitis nodularis helicis.

FEATURES (p. 18–19)

Benign

Incidence

Not common

Site

Pinna, usually at upper pole of helix

Clinical features (Figure 4.20)

- Commonest in men over 40
- Very painful nodule (0.5–1 cm diameter) on pinna, often with surrounding redness
- Usually occurs on side on which patient sleeps; pain interferes with sleeping

ACCEPTABLE MANAGEMENT

- Simple measures to relieve pressure on helix while awaiting surgery
- Excision of nodule with small margin of normal skin
- Refer for surgery if lesion large or diagnosis difficult

RECOMMENDED TREATMENT

Excision

TREATMENT TO AVOID

Cryotherapy – this causes exquisite pain and is not effective

CAUTIONARY NOTES

Squamous cell carcinoma on the pinna can sometimes mimic chondrodermatitis nodularis helicis and vice versa

SOLAR KERATOSIS
SYNONYM Actinic keratosis, senile keratosis

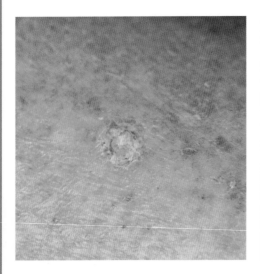 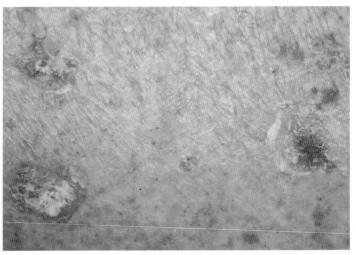

Figure 4.21 **(a)** Solar keratosis **(b)** Multiple solar keratoses.

FEATURES (p. 19–20)

Most benign; malignant transformation rare

Incidence

Common

Site

Light-exposed skin, e.g. backs of hands, face, scalp and ears

Clinical features (Figure 4.21)

- Caused by exposure to sunlight
- Commonest in fair-skinned elderly individuals
- Pink, scaly or warty lesions, usually less than 1.5 cm diameter
- Often multiple
- May be asymptomatic, sometimes itches
- May present as cutaneous horn
- Regresses in winter

ACCEPTABLE MANAGEMENT

- Referral if diagnostic uncertainty
- Leave alone if confident of diagnosis; warn patient to return if lesion changes
- Give advice about sun protection
- Cryotherapy – must be confident of diagnosis as no histological confirmation; hypopigmented scar may result
- Curettage and cautery – warn about possible scarring; histological confirmation from curettings

RECOMMENDED TREATMENT

- Leave alone; warn patient to return if lesion changes
- Cryotherapy (p. 120–23) if diagnosis is confident

TREATMENT TO AVOID

Ellipse excision

CAUTIONARY NOTES

Refer if suspect squamous cell carcinoma

BOWEN'S DISEASE

SYNONYM Intra-epithelial squamous cell carcinoma, intra-epidermal carcinoma *in situ*

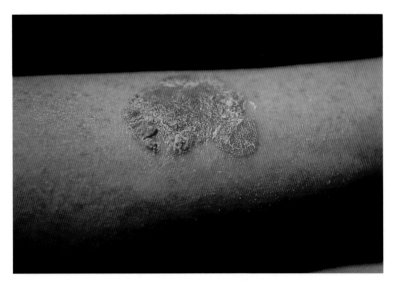

Figure 4.22 Bowen's disease.

FEATURES (p. 20–21)
Premalignant

Incidence
Quite common

Site
Lower legs

Clinical features (Figure 4.22)
- Commonest in elderly
- Persistent scaly erythematous plaque
- Differential diagnosis is eczema, psoriasis, tinea corporis – failure to respond to topical treatment may be a useful diagnostic clue
- Progression to squamous cell carcinoma inevitable; may take many years

ACCEPTABLE MANAGEMENT
- Refer
- If patient frail, consider biopsy of plaque followed by staged cryotherapy (p. 120–23)

RECOMMENDED TREATMENT
Refer

TREATMENT TO AVOID
Extensive surgical excision – healing on lower limb in elderly is often poor

CAUTIONARY NOTES
Following transformation to squamous cell carcinoma, rapid enlargement and spread likely

KERATOACANTHOMA
SYNONYM Molluscum sebaceum

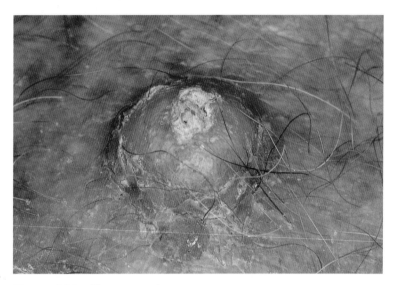

Figure 4.23 Keratoacanthoma.

FEATURES (p. 21–22)

Benign, but difficult to differentiate from squamous cell carcinoma

Incidence

Less common than basal cell or squamous cell carcinoma

Site

Commonest on light-exposed skin

Clinical features (Figure 4.23)
- Rapidly enlarging lesion over 6–8 weeks
- Symmetrical pink nodule 10–20 mm in diameter; central crater filled with keratin plug
- Spontaneous resolution occurs
- Histologically indistinguishable from squamous cell carcinoma; preoperative appearance vital in making diagnosis

ACCEPTABLE MANAGEMENT

Urgent referral

RECOMMENDED TREATMENT

Urgent referral

TREATMENT TO AVOID

Do not leave to resolve spontaneously

CAUTIONARY NOTES

Beware the undiagnosed squamous cell carcinoma

LENTIGO MALIGNA
SYNONYM Hutchinson's freckle

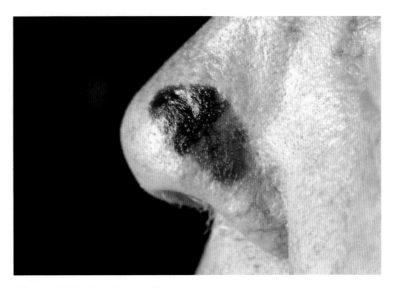

Figure 4.24   Lentigo maligna.

FEATURES (p. 22)
Premalignant

Incidence
Not rare; much less common than solar keratosis

Site
Face, usually upper cheek, temple or forehead

Clinical features (Figure 4.24)
- Usually occurs in 60–70-year-olds
- Flat, brown 'stain'-like appearance
- Slowly enlarging over many years
- Gradually becomes darker, with marked variation in colour
- Can eventually develop a nodule, indicating transformation to invasive lentigo maligna melanoma

ACCEPTABLE MANAGEMENT
Refer

RECOMMENDED TREATMENT
Refer

TREATMENT TO AVOID
Cryotherapy – atypical melanocytic proliferation will recur after this treatment

CAUTIONARY NOTES
Differential diagnosis basal cell papilloma. Do not underestimate risk of progression to invasive lentigo maligna melanoma

BASAL CELL CARCINOMA
SYNONYM Rodent ulcer

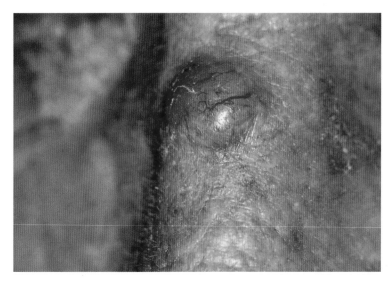

Figure 4.25 Basal cell carcinoma.

FEATURES (p. 23–25)

Locally malignant

Incidence

Commonest skin cancer in white-skinned people; related to sun exposure

Site

Light-exposed sites, particularly the face

Clinical features (Figure 4.25)

- Slowly enlarging, non-healing lesion; sometimes ulcerated, sometimes scabbed
- Nodulocystic is commonest type
- Cystic, pearly appearance with superficial telangiectasia
- Locally invasive, said not to metastasize
- Other variants less common, i.e. pigmented, morphoeic, superficial

ACCEPTABLE MANAGEMENT

- Refer for diagnosis and treatment
- Consider complete surgical excision and regular follow-up for a frail, elderly patient with a small lesion (p. 40)

RECOMMENDED TREATMENT

Refer

TREATMENT TO AVOID

Cryotherapy – this is only of value for superficial basal cell carcinomas, which are uncommon and more difficult to diagnose

CAUTIONARY NOTES

- Look for the second BCC or other skin cancers
- Morphoeic basal cell carcinomas difficult to remove completely

SQUAMOUS CELL CARCINOMA

SYNONYM Epidermoid carcinoma

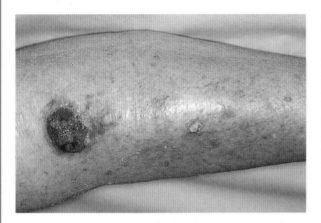 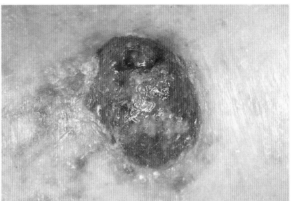

Figure 4.26 **(a)** Squamous cell carcinoma arising from a patch of Bowen's disease on the leg **(b)** Close up of the squamous cell carcinoma seen in **(a)**.

FEATURES (p. 25–26)

Malignant

Incidence

Less common than basal cell carcinomas, much commoner than malignant melanoma; related to sun exposure

Site

Sun-damaged skin of elderly

Clinical features (Figure 4.26)

- Indurated, crusted, keratotic plaque
- May develop into non-healing ulcer with irregular raised edge
- Can arise in Bowen's disease on lower limbs of elderly
- Much more malignant than basal cell carcinomas; lymphatic spread and metastatic disease occur

ACCEPTABLE MANAGEMENT

Refer

RECOMMENDED TREATMENT

Refer

TREATMENT TO AVOID

- Inadequate surgical excision
- Cryotherapy

CAUTIONARY NOTES

Combined approach between dermatologists, plastic surgeons and radiotherapists may be necessary

MALIGNANT MELANOMA

SYNONYM None

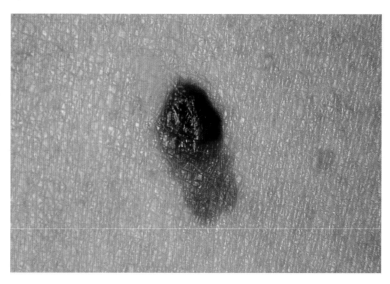

Figure 4.27 Malignant melanoma.

FEATURES (p. 26–28)

Malignant

Incidence

Doubled in last 10 years but still less common than other types of skin cancer; female:male 2:1.

Site

Commoner on lower legs of women and trunk of men

Clinical features (Figure 4.27)

- Superficial spreading malignant melanoma is commonest (80%)
- Others rare, e.g. nodular, acral, amelanotic
- 70% arise *de novo*, 30% in pre-existing moles
- Suspicious features in pigmented lesion: change in size, shape or colour
- Prognosis excellent for thin tumours diagnosed early, poor for thick tumours diagnosed late

ACCEPTABLE MANAGEMENT

Refer

RECOMMENDED TREATMENT

Refer

TREATMENT TO AVOID

Managing it yourself – you cannot be expected to have up-to-date knowledge of management and prognosis

CAUTIONARY NOTES

- Refer suspicious pigmented lesions urgently
- Don't panic if you remove a melanoma; discuss histology report with an expert and decide on management before you speak to the patient

Part Two

Facilities and Skills

Chapter 5
Background information

This chapter outlines the resources you need to carry out minor operations. The procedures described in this book require few special facilities: a suitable room, a couch or operating table and adequate lighting. New equipment is expensive but second-hand equipment from hospitals or other suppliers is perfectly serviceable and much cheaper. Comprehensive record keeping is vital for good patient care and audit as well as for medicolegal reasons.

FACILITIES

Equipment requirements

MINOR SURGERY ROOM

You need a room suitable for minor operations. A treatment room is usually adequate. Hand washing facilities are essential and the floor covering must be easy to clean. A bright, adjustable light with a focused beam is essential. It can be free-standing or fixed to the ceiling.

An examination couch is usually adequate, although an adjustable-height operating table with head-down tilt makes operating safer and more comfortable. An adjustable stool helps with delicate procedures, and an arm-board attached to the side of the table is useful for operations on the upper limb. You should be able to walk around the table freely: if it is against a wall you may have difficulty managing an emergency (Figure 5.1).

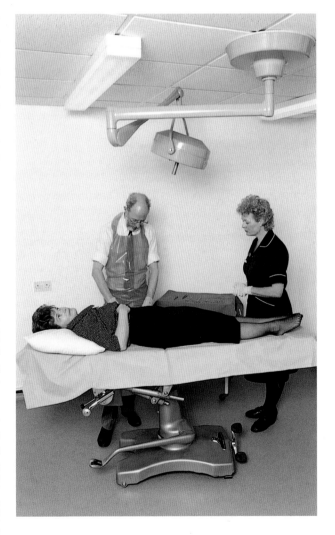

Figure 5.1 A suitably equipped minor surgery room.

BASIC REQUIREMENTS FOR INFECTION CONTROL

Hand washing

You must have a wash basin with a dispenser for liquid soap and paper towels. There is no place for a slimy bar of soap in a dish or a cloth towel hanging on the wall.

Skin preparation

Single-use disposable sterile dressing packs which contain all you need for each procedure are now available. Use an aqueous-based antiseptic solution in single-use sachets.

Sterilization

A bench-top autoclave is essential unless you have an alternative supply of sterile instruments. You should have a dirty sink where instruments can be washed (see p. 79 for details).

Miscellaneous

High quality sterile disposable latex gloves are essential, as are facilities for safe disposal of sharps and clinical waste. A trolley is useful for setting out instruments and dressing packs. Disposable plastic aprons help to protect clothing. Gowns and masks are unnecessary (see p. 78).

EQUIPMENT FOR SURGICAL PROCEDURES

Local anaesthesia

You will need different sizes of disposable syringes and needles, together with supplies of local anaesthetic agents. Consider buying a dental syringe, with disposable needles and single-use vials of lignocaine. See Chapter 6 for details.

Instruments

Carefully think through each procedure and plan your instruments accordingly. If you are going to operate on a number of patients in a session you will need several sets of instruments in order to avoid waiting for them to come out of the autoclave.

Surgical instruments are delicate and expensive. Cheap, poor quality instruments are a false economy since they soon start to fail. For example, needle-holders slip and forceps do not meet. This becomes intensely irritating. Buy the best you can afford and look after them. Do not store ratchet instruments, e.g. needle-holders and artery forceps, with the ratchet fully closed but keep them on the first notch to prevent overstraining the hinge.

There follows a list of recommended instruments. Each type is available in many versions. In practice the differences do not matter much.

A basic set of instruments is as follows (Figure 5.2):

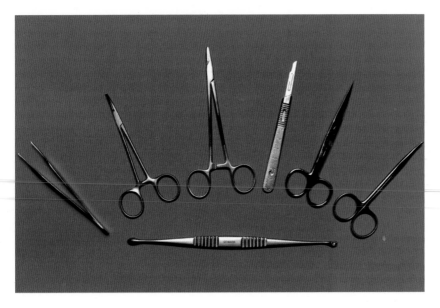

Figure 5.2 Essential instruments. (Reproduced by permission of Seward Medical Ltd.)

- scalpel handle size 3 with disposable No. 15 blades;
- strabismus scissors (curved) 4.5 in – for dissecting;
- dressing scissors (straight) 5 in – for cutting sutures;
- needle-holder (Crile Wood 14 cm);
- dissecting forceps (Adson 5 in – toothed and non-toothed);
- artery forceps (Halstead mosquito 5 in– curved on flat);
- curette (Volkman scoop 8.5 in).

The following additional instruments are extremely useful (Figure 5.3):
- skin hook (McIndoe single 7.5 in);
- catspaw retractor (Kilner 6 in);
- tissue forceps (Allis 6 in);
- large flat blades for shave excision.

Detailed information about the use of the instruments is contained in Chapter 7.

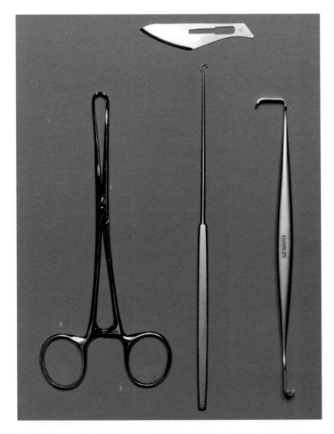

Figure 5.3 Desirable instruments. (Reproduced by permission of Seward Medical Ltd.)

Sutures

Have a range of sutures available. Become familiar with using a small selection, e.g.:
- Prolene or Ethilon monofilament 1.5 metric (4/0) – excellent for most skin closures;
- Prolene or Ethilon monofilament 2 metric (3/0) – good for subcuticular closures;
- Vicryl 2 metric (3/0) – good for subcuticular closures;
- Prolene or Ethilon monofilament 0.7 metric (6/0) – very fine suture, useful for fine facial work and in children.

Silk sutures should generally be avoided since they produce unsightly scars. However they can be useful on the scalp. Further information about the use of sutures is contained in Chapter 7.

Other equipment

Cryosurgical or electrocautery equipment. A rechargeable electrocautery unit is particularly useful. See Chapter 8 for details.

RESUSCITATION EQUIPMENT

All staff must know where the resuscitation equipment is kept. It should be marked clearly. Make sure it is checked regularly and that the drugs are all in date.

Staff

A trained nurse is invaluable to assist at procedures. In addition, he or she can be asked to deal with the instruments and supplies and the day-to-day running of the service. In large practices a member of the administrative staff may be helpful in booking operating sessions and in managing the paperwork.

Make sure you are fully aware of your responsibilities to your staff. You should have a written accident procedure and an incident book. See pp. 80 and 81 for further details.

RECORD KEEPING

It is sound clinical practice to keep written records of every minor procedure carried out. What system you use does not matter as long as it is effective and foolproof. It may be simply a combination of clinical notes and a minor procedure book. In addition, a computerized disease index and recall may be used.

Records are extremely important for medicolegal

reasons. Many problems arise years after the actual procedure was carried out. Without accurate written records it may be impossible to defend yourself against a claim, however unjust. Moreover, accurate record keeping is a condition of service and records are required when making claims for payment.

Information

Information required:
- patient's details (including contact telephone number);
- clinical diagnosis;
- whether urgent or routine;
- date of initial consultation;
- date of procedure;
- details of procedure – local anaesthetic (strength, type, with or without adrenaline), suture material and number of sutures;
- name of surgeon;
- whether specimen sent for histology;
- date the report was received, and any consequent action;
- final diagnosis;
- any postoperative complications;
- if patient is referred: urgent or routine, date of referral, and to whom.

Histology reports

You must record the dates on which specimens have been sent to the laboratory and be able to identify any for which a result has not been received within a specified time. Only by doing this will you avoid the possible disaster of overlooking an unexpected malignancy.

Your system should ensure that histology reports are seen by the doctor who carried out the procedure and who is responsible for any necessary further action. This is especially important in a large group practice.

Procedure book

The doctor or nurse should record a brief description of the procedure in the book. Details of the procedure, sutures inserted and local anaesthetic used, including batch numbers and expiry dates, may be recorded here or in the patient's notes.

It is useful to have one column to record specimens sent for histological examination and another to tick when the report comes back. Gaps in the latter column highlight missing reports.

A specially designed form may be used instead

(Figure 5.4). The information from these forms can easily be processed and, if appropriate, entered on to a computer system for analysis.

AUDIT

Self-criticism is vital if you are to keep improving your clinical work. The essence of audit is to examine an area of your practice and compare it with the standards to which you aspire. If your performance does not meet the standards, you should make the necessary changes and then re-examine the same area to confirm that your performance has improved. Without audit, it is easy to assume that all is well. Although this may be so, you cannot be sure unless you look.

It is important to know how often you remove malignant lesions, especially unexpected ones. Patient satisfaction too should be monitored systematically, since information in this area is often incomplete. For example, it may seem that your patients never get wound infections, simply because they never report them. However there may be other reasons for this: they may get infections which resolve spontaneously, or they may consult one of your partners for follow-up. It can be salutary to review patients 2 or 3 weeks after surgery.

The audit cycle is a constant process. By continually scrutinizing your own practice you will continue to improve it.

INFECTION CONTROL

You should be aware of the need for infection control at all times. Look critically at your own practice with this in mind. For each procedure you should choose the most suitable approach for controlling infection and consider who needs to be involved.

Monitor the infection rate in your practice. The Infection Control Department at your local hospital will be able to give useful guidance.

Hygiene

HAND WASHING

Hands are the most important source of cross-infection. Many people do not wash their hands adequately.

LOVEMEAD GROUP PRACTICE	Ref No:
Minor Surgery Information Sheet	Ref Date: / /

Patient Details

Surname:

Forename(s):

Address:

Telephone (Home):

Telephone (Work):

Date of Birth: / /   Normal GP:

Referring GP:

Consent Signed?

Provisional Diagnosis:

Proposed Operation: Site: Duration: mins   Urgent?   Venue:

Procedure Details

Appt Sent: / /   Booked Date: / /   Booked Time: :   Op Date: / /   Reason for Difference:

Operation Performed:

Performed by: FHSA Eligible?

Anaesthetic: Adrenalin?   Spec sent?   Specimen sent to:

Closure: Suture Size: Rmv Sutures in: days   Follow-up Date:

Details of Procedure:

Post-op Assessment:
- [ ] Bleeding
- [ ] Wound Infection
- [ ] Wound Breakdown
- [ ] Unsightly Scarring

Histology Details

Date Spec Sent: / /   Date Rpt Rec'd: / /   Date Seen by GP: / /   GP's Signature: Malignant?   Exc Comp?

Final Diagnosis:

Follow-up Action:

Form MS01   ©1994 The Philip Tilson Partnership   Rev 10 Mar-94

Figure 5.4   Minor procedure form, designed by one of the authors and used in his practice. (Reproduced by permission of the Philip Tilson Partnership, © The Philip Tilson Partnership 1994.)

Two kinds of bacterial flora affect the skin: resident and transient. The resident bacteria live deep in the skin and cannot be removed. Scrubbing the skin in an attempt to get rid of them only makes matters worse by bringing them to the surface.

Transient bacteria colonize the skin surface. They are picked up very easily but they can be removed equally easily by simple washing with liquid soap and water. After washing you may also use an alcohol-based antibacterial hand rubbing preparation.

Many studies have shown that even when people wash their hands carefully they often omit parts, especially in the skin creases and the areas between the fingers. Wash your hands scrupulously using an antiseptic solution and plenty of warm running water. Wetting your hands thoroughly before applying the handwash will reduce the likelihood of your hands getting sore. Dry your hands carefully with disposable paper towels, which may be sterile or not, depending on the procedure. Finally, apply an alcohol-based hand rub and let it dry completely.

Disposable paper towels are essential. It is well worth buying good-quality disposable paper towels or your hands may become sore with repeated drying. Communal cloth towels should never be used as they are extremely efficient at spreading infection.

PROTECTIVE CLOTHING

Sterile gloves should always be worn for the procedures described in this book. There is no need to wear a gown or mask since there is no evidence that these affect infection rates. A disposable plastic apron, however, provides useful protection. To avoid droplet infection, keeping your mouth shut by not talking is much more effective than wearing a mask!

CLEANING THE PATIENT'S SKIN

Elaborate skin preparation is unnecessary. Infection in general practice is uncommon and the cross-infection that bedevils hospitals is much less of a problem.

For most straightforward skin procedures simple cleaning with an alcohol-based antiseptic preparation is adequate. Any of the standard proprietary solutions is satisfactory. These contain antibacterial agents such as chlorhexidine or povidone-iodine. To be effective, alcohol-based solutions must be left to dry completely before carrying out the procedure.

Never use spirit with electrocautery, since this may produce severe burns.

It is usually unnecessary to shave the patient. If you are operating on a particularly hairy area, e.g. the scalp, remove the surrounding hair with sharp scissors or a clipper. Shaving large areas is unnecessary: it traumatizes the skin, encourages infection, and is unsightly and uncomfortable for the patient. Above all, never shave the eyebrows – they may not grow back!

Sterilization

DEFINITIONS

Decontamination

A general term covering methods of cleaning, disinfection and sterilization.

Disinfection

Inactivation of viruses, fungi and vegetative bacteria, but not necessarily bacterial spores.

Sterilization

Complete destruction or removal of microorganisms and their spores.

The skin is the main defence against infection. Any organism, even if it is normally of low pathogenicity, can cause infection if it breaches this barrier.

> *Golden rule:* When carrying out procedures that breach the patient's skin, you must use sterile instruments.

In the past 'sterilization' was sometimes rather hit and miss. Old fashioned methods such as boiling up instruments in hot water, using a domestic pressure cooker or soaking instruments in chemicals are dangerously unreliable. They are now totally unacceptable.

Sterile instruments may be obtained as follows.
- Use a bench-top autoclave. This is by far the best method. The only drawback is cost.
- Arrange to have your instruments sterilized by the local Central Sterile Supplies Department. Instruments are delivered in sterile packs.
- Buy disposable instruments and discard them after a single use.

AUTOCLAVES

Autoclaves work on the pressure cooker principle. They sterilize by transferring the latent heat of condensation to microorganisms on the surface of instruments. It is therefore essential that the autoclave is properly loaded so that the steam can get to all the surfaces of all the instruments. Bench-top autoclaves are ideal for GPs who do a lot of minor surgery (Figure 5.5).

The temperature, pressure and length of time the instruments stay in the autoclave are crucial for achieving sterilization. The machine monitors its own performance and has built-in quality controls.

Choose your autoclave carefully and make sure that whoever uses it knows exactly how to operate it and keeps a written record of each sterilizing cycle. Autoclaves must be operated according to the manufacturer's instructions and serviced regularly, usually by the supplier.

When choosing an autoclave make sure that:
• it meets the necessary British Standard specifications;
• it has chamber temperature and pressure indicators;
• it has an automatic cycle with an operating cycle indicator;
• it has a fault indicator.

An autoclave is only effective if instruments are free from any organic matter. All instruments must be clean before being sterilized. After use instruments should be scrubbed with a brush and detergent under running water in a separate sink from that used for hand washing.

Since this may cause a spray of dirty material, make sure that whoever does this job is properly protected with gloves and apron and, if necessary, eye protection. Scrubbing instruments under water reduces the spray.

The autoclave must be loaded properly with instruments laid out on special trays to enable steam to reach every surface (Figure 5.6).

It is important to follow the manufacturer's instructions concerning the use of distilled water.

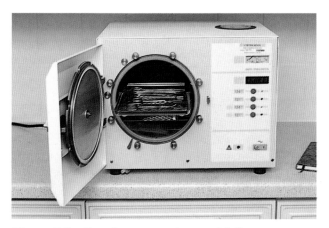

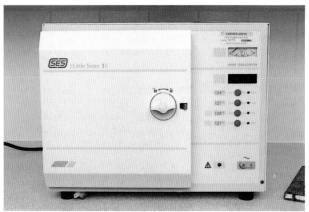

Figure 5.5 Bench-top autoclave. **(a)** Open. **(b)** Closed.

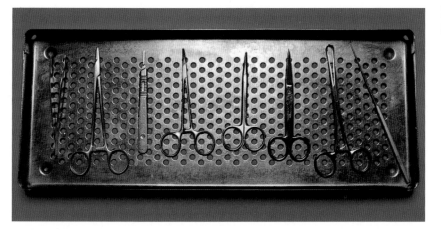

Figure 5.6 Sterilizing tray for bench-top autoclave.

Ordinary water may cause instruments to discolour permanently and corrode.

Ideally, instruments should be used as soon as they have cooled. However, if covered with sterile paper they can be used for up to 3 hours. You can sterilize several trays at once and use them for a number of patients in a session.

Bench-top autoclaves will not sterilize instruments in packets. Salesmen will sometimes try to persuade you that a bench-top autoclave will sterilize wrapped instruments in special sealed packets. This is not true. Only large autoclaves of the kind found in a hospital Central Sterile Supplies Department can do this.

OTHER METHODS OF STERILIZATION

Central Sterile Supplies Department (CSSD)

For doctors who only carry out occasional procedures an alternative to the expensive autoclave is the use of prepacked sterile instruments.

The CSSD at your local hospital will usually be able to supply you with such instruments in packs. You may choose to buy your own instruments or to hire them from the hospital, depending on local arrangements. Hospital instruments, however, are sometimes unsatisfactory: some are blunt or otherwise in poor condition. Sometimes the instruments supplied are different from those requested, which can be intensely irritating. Despite this, it is worth discussing your requirements with the CSSD before deciding whether to buy your own instruments and autoclave.

Disposable instruments

Disposable instruments, although expensive, can be useful for certain procedures. Scalpels, for example, are now available as disposable items.

Hot air sterilizers

Hot air sterilizers are ovens that sterilize by dry heat. This process takes much longer than using pressurized steam because the machines are slow to heat up and cool down. Unless they are fan-assisted they tend to create hot and cold spots inside the oven. In addition, the time needed for sterilization varies with the number of instruments. Although these machines can provide adequate sterilization, they are inconvenient and difficult to use safely, and are therefore not recommended. If you can afford it, an autoclave is a far better investment.

Infection control policy

Every practice should have a written infection control policy for all its staff. This should designate particular tasks to appropriate members of the practice team.

HEPATITIS B AND HUMAN IMMUNODEFICIENCY VIRUS (HIV)

The only safe policy is to assume that all patients may be positive for HIV or hepatitis B. The precautions required should depend on your assessment of the proposed procedure, not on your perception of the patient.

All staff involved in minor surgery should be immunized against hepatitis B. It is important that doctors and nurses keep up to date with guidelines on dealing with spillages of potentially infective material.

NEEDLESTICK INJURIES

These can be reduced to a minimum by following simple guidelines.
- Take care when performing surgery.
- Never resheath needles.
- Dispose of sharps in approved containers.

You should have a written procedure on what to do following a needlestick injury. The Microbiology or Infection Control Department at your local hospital will provide invaluable advice on this subject.

An excellent guide to infection control is published by the British Medical Association (see p. 129).

MEDICOLEGAL CONSIDERATIONS

Most medicolegal problems stem from poor communication. By ensuring that the patient understands fully the proposed procedure you will avoid many pitfalls.

Most of the procedures described in this book are fairly straightforward. Whenever you carry out a procedure, however, you must be able to demonstrate that you have the necessary knowledge and expertise. You should bear this in mind if you are asked to carry out a procedure of which you have insufficient experience.

CONSENT

Before performing any surgery take time to explain it carefully. Make sure the patient is aware of possible alternative treatments, e.g. a different surgical technique or continued observation.

Always warn the patient that any operation will result in a scar. Patients often do not realize this until after the operation. It is helpful to point out exactly where, and how long, the scar will be. Explain about the local anaesthetic and what your patient can expect to feel. This explanation must always be given by a doctor and should not be delegated.

The consensus from the medical defence bodies is that signed consent from the patient is not necessary, since he or she is giving implicit consent by attending for the operation. Moreover a signature on a standard consent form is no real safeguard. Nevertheless you need to be able to show that you have explained your intentions adequately, and that the patient's consent was fully informed and freely given. For this reason a written record that you have obtained consent is essential. Although a short descriptive entry in the patient's notes is adequate, the authors recommend the use of a consent form as shown in Figure 5.7.

Consent for minors

In general avoid operating on children, especially small ones. However calm they may seem in your consulting room they are apt to go berserk when faced with a needle. Sometimes it may be necessary to carry out a procedure on a patient under 16. In these circumstances you should obtain the parent's written consent. Occasionally this may not be possible. Provided you are satisfied that the patient is able to understand the procedure and its implications, and that he or she consents freely, you may decide to proceed. This decision will depend on the merits of the individual case. Remember that, as highlighted in the Children's Act 1989, children of all ages need to be party to the consenting process to an extent dependent upon their age.

RECORDS

It is essential to keep adequate written records of every procedure you perform. See pp. 75–76 for further details.

WRITTEN INFORMATION

Patients often forget what they are told, and it is useful to give them written information, both before and after the procedure, to reinforce what you have said. In particular, you may want to give patients a leaflet after an operation outlining what to expect, what to do if things go wrong and the date of a review appointment.

MISHAPS

Occasionally something will go wrong. If this happens, always contact your defence organization at once. It is common sense and courtesy to explain to your patient what has occurred and to apologize for any distress that may have been caused. The defence organisations recommend that you tell the patient the facts, but that you should not comment or speculate on the actions of others.

HEALTH AND SAFETY AT WORK

For most minor procedures you will be working with other members of staff, especially nurses. You have responsibilities as an employer as well as a doctor. You should therefore provide information, training and supervision to ensure the health and safety of practice ancillary staff. Be aware of the Health and Safety at Work Act 1974 and the Control of Substances Hazardous to Health Act 1988 (COSHH).

A clear written safety policy should be available for all employees. This should include arrangements for disposal of sharps and clinical waste. Every employer is legally required to keep an accident book on the premises. Make sure you are familiar with your obligations and that you keep up to date with changes, especially new European Union requirements.

IMPORTANT!

Please read this form very carefully. It contains important information about your proposed operation.

If there is anything you don't understand, or any points that you would like to know more about, you should ask your doctor now.

Please make sure that all the details about you on the form are correct. If they are, and you understand the explanations you have been given, then sign the form at the bottom.

For completion by the Doctor:

• I confirm that I have explained the procedure to be carried out, known as

....

to my patient, ... on .... (date).

• I have discussed the reasons for the procedure and the possible forms of treatment available.

• I have explained the kind of anaesthetic to be used, the procedure itself and the likely implications of these for the patient.

Signed: .... (General Practitioner) .... (date)

For completion by the Patient or Parent/Guardian:

• I understand that the procedure will be carried out by a General Practitioner.

• I have had the procedure and the anaesthesia explained to me and what their effects are likely to be, and I understand these explanations.

• I wish the procedure to be carried out and I confirm that I give my consent.

• I also consent to any further or alternative operative measures which may become necessary during the course of the procedure.

Signed: .... (Patient or Parent/Guardian) .... (date)

Figure 5.7 Example of a consent form used by one of the authors.

Chapter 6

Practical skills: anatomical hazards, local anaesthesia

ANATOMICAL HAZARDS AND PITFALLS

When carrying out the procedures described in this book you are unlikely to encounter deep-seated structures. However, some important structures, particularly nerves, lie just under the skin and these are at risk of damage during seemingly minor surgery.

Revise the anatomy of the area before starting, bearing in mind that many structures are variable in position. Remain observant throughout the procedure. Exercise particular caution when operating on the face.

There are certain notorious areas of the body where wounds tend to form bad scars or keloid. Other sites are particularly liable to poor healing. Surgery in these areas should be avoided if possible since the results are often disappointing. If surgery is unavoidable the patient should be warned of the likely results.

IMPORTANT ANATOMICAL STRUCTURES CLOSE TO THE SURFACE

Face

- **Mandibular branch of the facial nerve.** This crosses the lower border of the mandible. Division causes permanent weakness of the lip.
- **Parotid gland.** An apparently simple cyst in this area may prove to be a parotid tumour.
- **Superficial temporal artery.** Because this lies

superficially it is easily cut causing profuse bleeding. Although this can be alarming, it is easily controlled by ligating the artery. Because the collateral circulation is excellent there is no danger of ischaemia.
- **Eyes.** The region around the eyes and nose can be hazardous. Only operate here if you have particular experience. However, chalazions are easy and safe to treat by incision and curettage.

These anatomical hazards are shown in Figure 6.1.

Anterior triangle of neck

There are many important structures lying superficially. **Avoid this area entirely.**

Posterior triangle of neck

This is also an extremely hazardous area. Structures here are close to the surface, easily damaged and variable in position. The **spinal accessory nerve** is at particular risk (Figure 6.2). Division of this nerve leads to shoulder drop.

Hand

- **Extensor tendons.** These run just under the thin skin on the dorsum of the fingers and hand. They are therefore at risk from both the scalpel and cryosurgery.
- **Palm.** Not only are the flexor tendons close to the skin but there is no slack at all in the palm of the hand. Never excise a lesion from the palm since the wound may prove impossible to close.

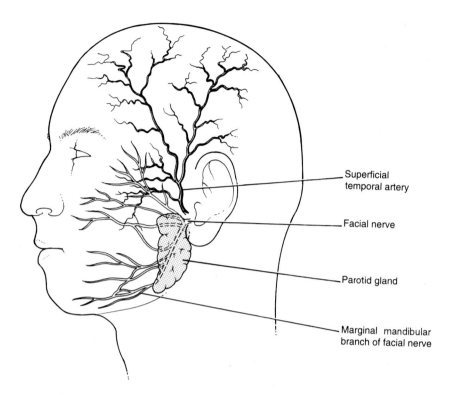

Superficial
temporal artery

Facial nerve

Parotid gland

Marginal mandibular
branch of facial nerve

Figure 6.1 The face, showing potential anatomical hazards.

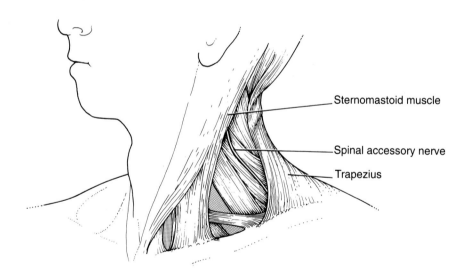

Sternomastoid muscle

Spinal accessory nerve

Trapezius

Figure 6.2 Posterior triangle of the neck.

Groin and axilla

Blood vessels and nerves. Avoid these areas altogether.

Lateral aspect of upper leg

Common peroneal (or lateral popliteal) nerve

(Figure 6.3). This is very superficial. Division of this nerve causes weakness of dorsiflexion of the foot.

Superficial nerves

Remember especially that lesions near superficial nerves may be neurofibromas.

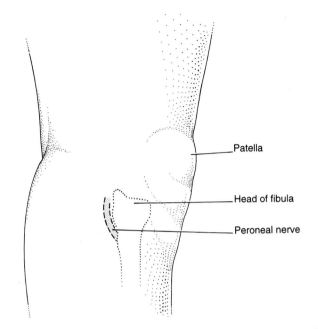

Figure 6.3 The common peroneal nerve at the knee.

AREAS PRONE TO SCARRING AND KELOID
FORMATION

- Sternum
- Shoulders

Wounds in these areas tend to form unsightly keloid scars, especially in people with pigmented skins. Moreover, these areas are usually exposed and are therefore best avoided altogether.

AREAS WHICH HEAL POORLY

Leg (anterior aspect)

This is especially so in the elderly. The skin overlying the subcutaneous border of the tibia is well known to heal slowly because its blood supply is poor. Avoid surgery here unless it is absolutely necessary.

Back

Wounds on the back heal slowly. Do not remove sutures too soon or the wound may open up.

LINES OF SKIN TENSION

Knowledge of the lines of skin tension is essential when planning any incision. See p. 94–5 for further details.

LOCAL ANAESTHESIA

Introduction

Most minor skin procedures require local anaesthesia, usually the injection of a local anaesthetic agent into the skin. However for a procedure to be successful the patient must feel confident that the doctor is fully in control of the situation.

Even with complete pain control patients may still be aware of pressure at the operation site. An anxious patient may perceive this sensation as pain. It is therefore vital to help the patient feel at ease.

- Establish a rapport.
- Make sure the patient fully understands the procedure and what it will involve.
- Develop a confident and reassuring manner.

Throughout the procedure you should remain aware of how the patient is reacting in order to spot problems, such as local anaesthetic toxicity, in their earliest stages.

INFORMATION

Patients often have a rather hazy idea of what is going to be done to them. However carefully you may have explained the procedure to them in advance, patients often fail to take in what has been said, or forget it. Keeping your patient fully informed of what is happening, and what you are going to do next, makes him or her feel much more confident.

It is especially important to warn patients about postoperative pain and how to deal with it. Consider advice on driving after the procedure, and whether someone should be with the patient for the first 24 hours or so. Written information about what to expect and what to do if problems arise can be very reassuring.

Anaesthetic agents

The most familiar is lignocaine. It is an effective and safe drug provided you understand its limitations.

Two longer-acting local anaesthetics are available: bupivacaine and prilocaine. However, they can cause problems such as methaemoglobinaemia and offer no particular advantage in most minor surgery.

DOSAGES

The maximum safe dosages for lignocaine quoted in the literature can be very misleading. Every patient should be assessed as an individual since the effect of a local anaesthetic depends on a number of factors, e.g. size of patient, tissue perfusion, presence of infection, cardiac output, drug distribution and metabolism.

> **Golden rule:** *you should be aware of the signs of over-dosage and act quickly if they occur.*

As a rule of thumb 3 mg/kg is widely used to calculate the maximum safe dose. So for an average 70 kg man, 210 mg of lignocaine could theoretically be used. The widely quoted 'maximum adult dose' of 200 mg corresponds to:
- 40 ml of 0.5% lignocaine solution
- 20 ml of 1% lignocaine solution
- 10 ml of 2% lignocaine solution.

In practice, for the sort of procedures described you will need only a few millilitres of local anaesthetic. But beware if you are treating multiple lesions at the same time, as the effects of each injection are cumulative.

PREPARATIONS

Lignocaine solution is available in three strengths; 0.5%, 1% and 2%. For most purposes 1% lignocaine is adequate. Each strength of lignocaine is also available with adrenaline 1:200 000 (see below).

Lignocaine solution is supplied in single-dose vials and multi-dose bottles. Although single-dose vials are slightly more expensive than multi-dose bottles, they are preferable because their use minimizes the risk of contamination

An alternative refinement is to use a dental syringe with a lignocaine cartridge (see below).

Adrenaline

Adrenaline is a double-edged sword.

The vasoconstriction produced by adrenaline can be an advantage: by reducing bleeding it makes procedures technically easier. This can be particularly useful for operations on the scalp. Adrenaline also reduces the systemic absorption of local anaesthetic, enabling larger volumes to be used without toxicity.

However, the vasoconstriction can also be a disadvantage: adrenaline in an end-artery causes intense vasospasm and may completely cut off the blood flow. If the collateral circulation is inadequate the territory of the affected artery will become ischaemic, with disastrous consequences.

> **Golden rule:** *never use local anaesthetic containing adrenaline when anaesthetizing any part of the body supplied by an end-artery (e.g. a digit, the penis, the tip of the nose).*

In our opinion, plain lignocaine is adequate for almost all the procedures we describe. If you avoid stocking solutions containing adrenaline there will be no possibility of confusion. However, many doctors do use adrenaline, and provided you are aware of the possible hazards it is perfectly safe.

Technique

ORDINARY SYRINGE

It is easiest to draw up the lignocaine using a green needle. When administering it, however, you should use the finest suitable needle to minimize the pain of the injection (usually an orange needle). Make sure that the local anaesthetic solution is not too cold, as this causes unnecessary pain.

DENTAL SYRINGE

You should consider buying a dental syringe. A disposable needle is screwed into the barrel of a metal syringe, and a sterile single-dose glass vial is inserted (Figure 6.4).

A variety of pre-packed local anaesthetic agents in different strengths is available. Sterility is no problem and the syringe is very convenient to use. Moreover, dental needles are finer than ordinary ones and produce much less discomfort. If you decide to buy a dental syringe you should also buy a special gadget for removing the used dental needle from the syringe.

Using a normal dental syringe it is not possible to draw back with the plunger in the conventional way. This might cause concern but in practice it is not a problem. Provided you keep the needle moving slowly and inject steadily, even if the point passes through a tiny vessel it will spend only a fraction of a second in the lumen. The amount of local anaesthetic reaching the bloodstream will be infinitesimal.

If you are particularly worried, it is in fact possible to aspirate with the dental syringe by pressing gently up and down on the plunger. Alternatively, specially designed self-aspirating dental syringes are available.

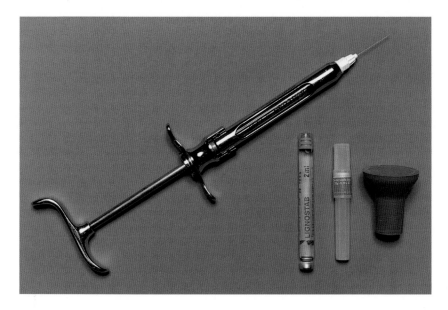

Figure 6.4 Dental syringe and needle, vial of local anaesthetic and needle remover.

LOCAL INFILTRATION

Confirm with your patient which lesion or lesions you are going to treat. In some cases it is advisable to mark the lesion with a marker pen (p. 110), particularly if it lies deep to the skin. It is highly embarrassing to find that a lesion has disappeared after you have infiltrated with local anaesthetic. Warn patients that as you start they will feel a sharp scratch which will soon subside.

For small lesions a fan-like approach, using two skin punctures at opposite sides of the lesion, is often sufficient (Figure 6.5(a)).

For larger lesions encircling is more appropriate. Anaesthetic is injected around the lesion, each time through skin that has already been numbed (Figure 6.5(b)). It is important to infiltrate all round the lesion and deep to it.

In vascular areas such as the scalp you should keep the number of puncture points to a minimum to reduce bleeding. If you are using a dental syringe with a long fine needle you will usually be able to manage with two punctures.

Although lignocaine works very quickly it is not instantaneous. If you do not allow enough time for it

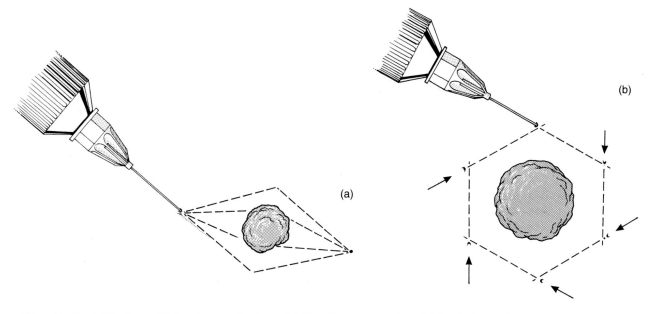

Figure 6.5 Infiltrating with local anaesthetic. **(a)** Fan-like approach. **(b)** Encirclement.

to take effect you will lose the patient's confidence. Explain that you are going to demonstrate that the injection is working. When you touch the skin with an instrument the patient should notice a difference between normal and anaesthetized skin. If he or she does not, give more anaesthetic until the patient is reassured that anaesthesia is complete.

RING BLOCK

This is a very useful technique for any procedure on a finger or toe.

Golden rules for ring blocks

Golden rule: never use a local anaesthetic containing adrenaline.

This can result in the loss of a finger or toe and is indefensible.

Golden rule: always wait long enough before starting the procedure.

Since the local anaesthetic effect takes some time to reach the distal end of the digit, resist the temptation to start too soon. Give the block, then go away and do something else while it takes effect.

Golden rule: never give ring blocks to patients with diabetes or peripheral vascular disease.

Golden rule: never inject local anaesthetic through infected skin.

Technique (Fig. 6.6)

The digital nerves run along each side of the digit close to the bone, but there are often additional twigs which run much more superficially.
1. Raise a bleb over the dorsum of the digit, just distal to the metacarpophalangeal or metatarsophalangeal joint, to anaesthetize the dorsal twigs of the digital nerves.
2. Angle the needle towards the palm or sole and inject about 0.5 ml of local anaesthetic along one side of the digit.
3. Withdraw the needle and inject similarly on the other side of the digit.

Beware of injecting too much fluid since this may cause pressure ischaemia. Usually 1—2 ml is all that is required — provided that you wait long enough for it to take effect.

Hazards

REACTIONS TO LOCAL ANAESTHETICS

The majority of so-called allergic reactions to local anaesthetic are in fact reactions to preservatives or other additives in the solution. True allergy is exceptionally rare. It is important always to ask patients if they have had problems with local anaesthetic injections in the past. Be aware of the rare but important conditions, such as porphyria, which are contraindications to the use of lignocaine.

OVERDOSAGE

The early symptoms and signs of lignocaine overdosage are circumoral tingling, tinnitus and slight

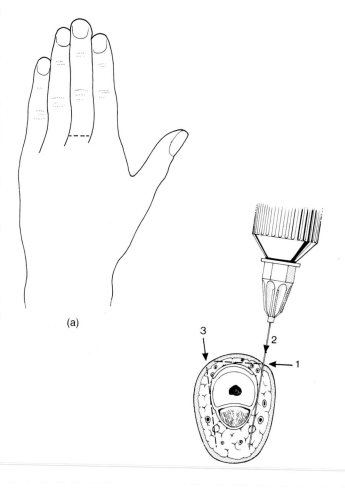

Figure 6.6 Ring block. **(a)** Injection site. **(b)** Technique – stages 1, 2, 3.

confusion or oddness of speech. Sometimes the patient will complain of a metallic taste. By talking to the patient you will notice these signs immediately and stop giving further anaesthetic.

If overdosage continues, the patient may develop nystagmus, dysphasia or muscular fasciculation. In later stages loss of consciousness supervenes, with fits, cardiac arrhythmias and respiratory and cardiac arrest.

RESUSCITATION

Fortunately serious problems are very uncommon. However, it is very important that everyone knows what to do if things go wrong and a patient collapses.

GET HELP

The first step is to get help. You will usually have a nurse or other assistant with you. If not, shout or telephone for immediate assistance.

ASSESSMENT

The commonest problem is a simple faint. It is important to diagnose and treat this promptly to avoid inappropriately aggressive resuscitative measures!

Sometimes a patient will collapse with a much more serious condition, e.g. a myocardial infarction or an anaphylactic reaction. It is vitally important that you have thought through in advance how to deal with this situation. You must also ensure that all your practice staff know what to do in an emergency.

PREVENTION

Planning

Contingency plans for dealing with unexpected collapse should be regularly rehearsed with all members of the practice team.

Equipment

Decide what equipment is required. This will depend on the sort of procedure you are proposing to do and on your local facilities. Some practices, for example, are within a few minutes' reach of a fully equipped ambulance staffed by highly trained paramedics. Others may be much more remote.

A minimum should probably be:
- cannulae, giving set and intravenous fluids (both colloid and crystalloid), including adhesive skin tape
- essential drugs, including adrenaline, hydrocortisone and chlorpheniramine
- airways
- oxygen, bag and face masks
- suction (mains or mechanically operated)
- laryngoscope and endotracheal tubes.

Ideally every practice should have the following:
- an ECG monitor
- a defibrillator.

Training

You must ensure that you are fully up to date with modern procedures and policies. Make sure you and your staff attend regular practical courses on cardiopulmonary resuscitation.

A summary of the current guidelines on cardiopulmonary resuscitation should be available in all rooms where minor procedures are carried out (Figure 6.7) illustrated on the next page.

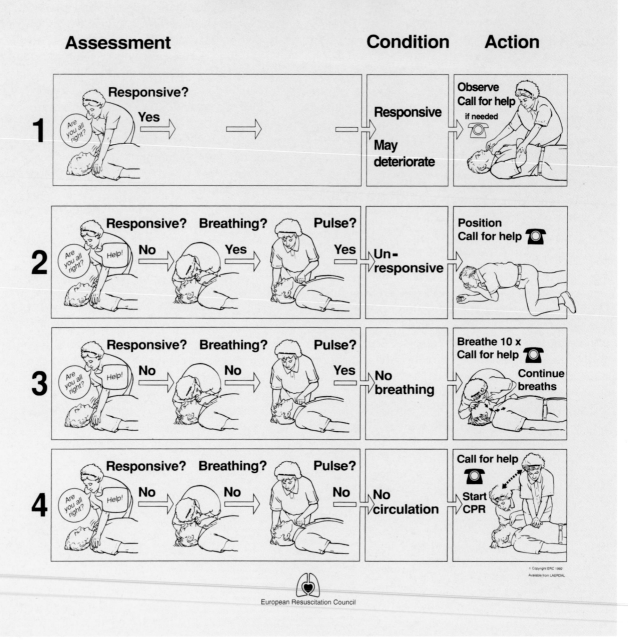

(a)

Figure 6.7 European Resuscitation Council guidelines for **(a)** basic and **(b)** advanced cardiac life support. (Reproduced by permission of the European Resuscitation Council, © European Resuscitation Council 1994).

ADVANCED CARDIAC LIFE SUPPORT

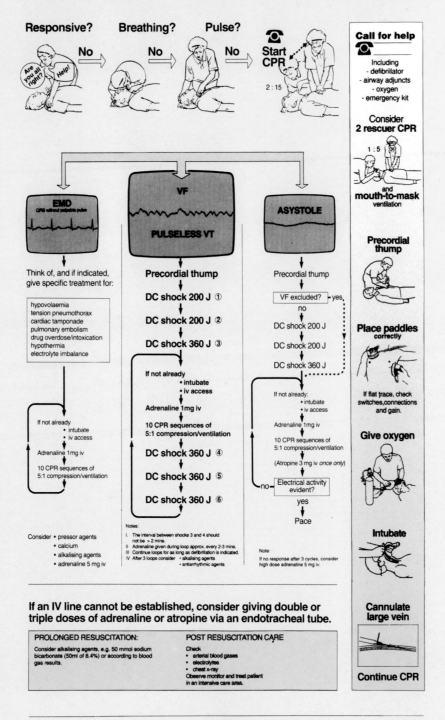

If an IV line cannot be established, consider giving double or triple doses of adrenaline or atropine via an endotracheal tube.

PROLONGED RESUSCITATION:	POST RESUSCITATION CARE
Consider alkalising agents, e.g. 50 mmol sodium bicarbonate (50ml of 8.4%) or according to blood gas results.	Check • arterial blood gases • electrolytes • chest x-ray Observe monitor and treat patient in an intensive care area.

European Resuscitation Council

(b)

Chapter 7

Practical skills: basic surgical technique

APPROACH

Certain principles are fundamental to all surgical procedures. Sound surgical technique makes the difference between a good and a bad result. This chapter concentrates on the techniques required to excise a lesion and sew up the wound neatly. A number of the points made may seen obvious, but they are worth making as many doctors have forgotten them by the time they take up minor surgery.

Other methods, e.g. cryosurgery, curettage and electrocautery are described in Chapter 8.

Aim

Patients may ask you to remove a skin lesion because of anxiety about cancer, because it looks ugly or because it gets in the way. Before you decide to excise a lesion you must be confident that you can remove it satisfactorily, allowing adequate margins in all directions, including deep to the lesion. You must also have a sound knowledge of wound healing so that you can achieve the best possible cosmetic result. Unless the result looks better than the original lesion the patient will be very unhappy.

Before removing a lesion you should carefully think the procedure through. If you fail to do this you may find yourself contemplating a wound with no clear idea of how best to close it.

Contingency plans

During a procedure you may occasionally find you are out of your depth: you may encounter structures which look important but which you cannot identify, a lesion may be deeper than anticipated, or you may cut a vessel by mistake and have to contend with bleeding obscuring your view.

When things do not go as expected stay calm and assess the situation. If the wound is bleeding profusely press it steadily with a swab and wait. This will always bring bleeding under control. Do not grab blindly with artery forceps. While you are waiting call for help – a partner can provide good retraction and give moral support.

Resist the temptation to go on with the procedure if things are really going wrong. Instead close the wound or cover it with a dressing, applying pressure if necessary. Then telephone a surgical colleague and ask advice. Nothing will suffer except your pride if someone more experienced has to redo the procedure a week or two later. Although such a situation is extremely unlikely, it is sensible to make sure that you have contacts with suitable colleagues whom you could call on for help.

Haemostasis

Severe bleeding is not usually a problem with the procedures described. Provided you select your lesions carefully you will not be operating near large blood vessels. Nevertheless, wounds often ooze alarmingly. Remember that a little blood goes a long way and bleeding usually looks worse than it is.

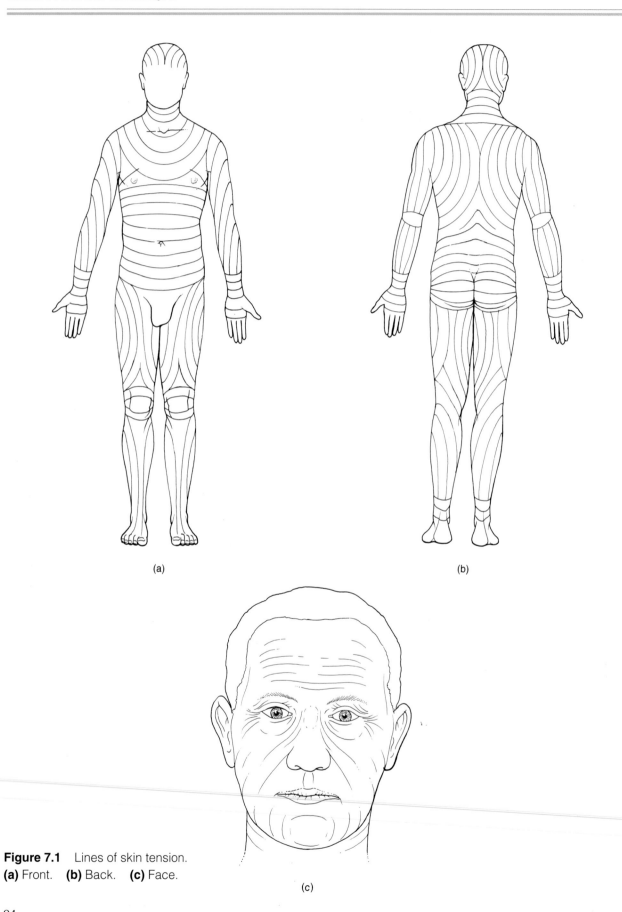

(a)

(b)

Figure 7.1 Lines of skin tension.
(a) Front.   **(b)** Back.   **(c)** Face.

(c)

Simple pressure with a swab is often all that is needed. Provided you press for long enough, most bleeding will stop. Cauterizing the wound with the ball-ended electrocautery burner is very helpful if the oozing continues. Occasionally you may need to ligate a small vessel by catching the bleeding end with artery forceps and tying it with fine catgut. Only catch a vessel if you can see it – clamping blindly is extremely dangerous.

Warn your patient before you begin if you think there may be excessive bleeding – patients find it disquieting if they suddenly see a lot of blood, especially if they think you did not expect it.

Incisions

SKIN CREASES

Skin creases are the key to good results. The skin naturally falls into creases according to the stresses acting upon it. These can be seen easily in the face, for example. They are more obvious in the elderly (Figure 7.1).

If your incision lies along or parallel to one of these lines, the edges will tend to come together naturally. If you fly in the face of these lines and site your incision across them, the wound's edges will tend to separate. Tight sutures will be needed to bring the edges together, resulting in swelling, ischaemia, poor healing and a nasty scar.

If you cannot see the natural creases try bunching up the skin. If you still cannot see creases it probably does not matter which way you make your incision. Avoid going across skin creases, especially over the flexor aspects of joints.

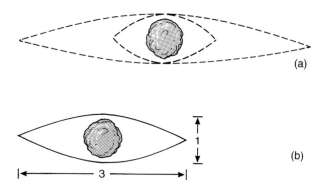

Figure 7.2 Ellipse excision. **(a)** Ellipse proportions. **(b)** Recommended proportions.

Elliptical incisions

If the lesion is in the skin itself, an ellipse of skin should be excised to achieve a neat scar; the longer the ellipse in relation to its width, the narrower the scar, but the greater its overall length (Figure 7.2(a)). As a general rule you should use a ratio of length:width of about 3:1 (Figure 7.2(b)).

Aim for a margin of excision of 2 mm. This will usually provide adequate clearance should the lesion unexpectedly prove to be malignant.

Linear incisions

If a lesion is entirely deep to the skin, make a linear incision. Then reach inside, dissect the lesion free and remove it. If you have designed the incision

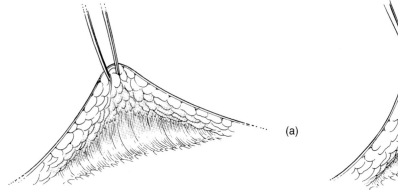

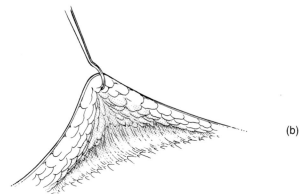

Figure 7.3 Handling the wound edge. **(a)** Using forceps. **(b)** Using a skin hook.

carefully along the natural lines of tension the edges of the wound should come together naturally. This is like opening a cupboard door, reaching inside for a jar of jam and then closing the door.

Do not make the mistake of trying to manage with a tiny incision. Such incisions make surgery difficult and may have to be extended, producing a worse result than if you had used an adequate incision in the first place.

Wound care

How well a wound heals depends on the blood supply to its edges, which in turn depends on your design and technique. Any tension in the suture line reduces blood supply, which may lead to infection and scarring.

Wound edges are very vulnerable and should be handled with great care. Even fine instruments can do a lot of damage although you may not see this with the naked eye. If possible avoid touching the skin edges with forceps but pick up the subcutaneous tissue instead (Figure 7.3(a)). Better still, use skin hooks (Figure 7.3(b)).

INSTRUMENTS AND HOW TO USE THEM

You only need a few instruments, but you should understand exactly how each works and what its limitations are. As with the prescription of drugs it is better to know a small number well than to use too many.

Handling instruments

To use any instrument requiring fine control your hand needs to be relaxed. This applies equally to using a pen, a violin bow or a pair of dissecting forceps. People frequently force their hands into contortions by holding surgical instruments wrongly.

The most relaxed position is midway between full pronation and full supination. After a short time at either extreme your hand will become tired and control will suffer. Once you become familiar with holding instruments correctly they become an extension of your hands.

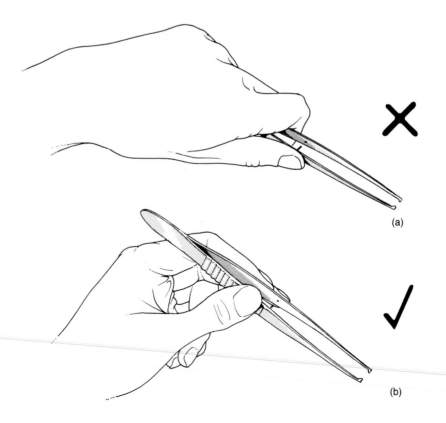

(a)

(b)

Figure 7.4 Holding forceps. **(a)** Incorrect method. **(b)** Correct method.

Types

Instruments fall into two main categories: **instruments for holding,** such as dissecting forceps, artery forceps, needle-holders and retractors, and **instruments for cutting,** such as scissors and scalpels.

INSTRUMENTS FOR HOLDING

Dissecting forceps

Dissecting forceps allow you to manipulate the tissue with one hand (usually the non-dominant one) while you do something else to it with the other – such as suturing. For fine control it is important to hold the forceps properly.

A surprising number of people automatically pick forceps up as shown in Figure 7.4(a). This forces the hand into full pronation, which quickly becomes very tiring. Instead, use them as shown in Figure 7.4(b):

Forceps may be toothed or non-toothed (Figure 7.5).

It is a mistake to think that non-toothed forceps can do no damage to the skin edge. In fact they can do more damage than the toothed variety if the jaws keep slipping off. Grasp the wound just deep to the edge, not actually on it.

Artery forceps and needle-holders

Artery forceps and needle-holders look superficially similar. They are in fact quite different. Although either may have curved or straight handles the crucial difference lies in the structure of the jaws.

- **Artery forceps** have delicate jaws. The surface of each has parallel grooves which coincide with those of the other jaw to form a series of circular channels when the instrument is closed (Figure 7.6).

   This design makes it possible to grasp tissue delicately without extensive crushing. However, if you try to hold a needle it will align itself along one of these channels and swivel round, making it impossible to put in a suture with precision (Figures 7.6, 7.7).

- **Needle-holders** have short powerful jaws. The surface of each jaw has criss-cross lines cut into it (Figure 7.8).

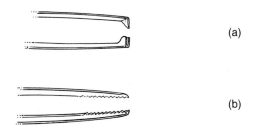

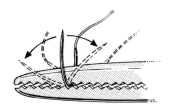

Figure 7.5 Dissecting forceps. **(a)** Toothed. **(b)** Non-toothed.

Figure 7.7 Needle aligning itself along grooves in artery forceps.

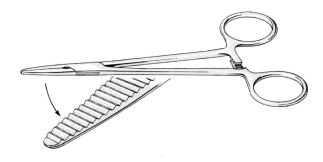

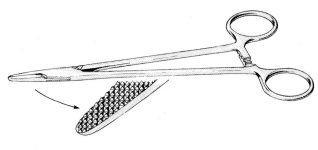

Figure 7.6 Artery forceps, showing detail of jaws.

Figure 7.8 Needle-holder, showing detail of jaws.

These jaws can grasp a needle firmly without it slipping round. However, if you use the instrument to pick up tissue, the jaws will crush it and cause damage.

Holding a needle

The central section of a needle is flattened and is designed to be grasped by the needle-holder. Hold the needle about two-thirds of the way from the point. If you hold it nearer the point you will be unable to take a decent bite before the needle-holder's jaws get in the way. If you are too far the other way the needle may buckle and snap.

Grasp the needle with the tip of the needle-holder. If the needle is too near the hinge, again the jaws will get in the way. It is useful to angle the needle slightly forward in the instrument's jaws. This makes the movement of inserting sutures more comfortable (Figure 7.9).

When you have positioned the needle in the needle-holder take your fingers out of the instrument's handles. Hold it in the palm of your hand when suturing, with your index finger along the handle to steady it. This position increases your range of movement and control (Figure 7.10).

INSTRUMENTS FOR CUTTING

Dissecting scissors

Dissecting scissors are curved and have blunt ends (Figure 7.11).

These may be used in the conventional way to cut tissue. In addition, the rounded points allow you to develop tissue planes by blunt dissection. By opening the scissors gently you can separate structures without harming them, provided there is a natural plane of cleavage (Figure 7.12). Often you can combine these two techniques. This is especially useful when dissecting an epidermoid cyst free from its surroundings (Figure 7.45).

The curvature of the scissors' blades allows you to hug the contours of a cyst while you are dissecting it. Dissecting scissors are delicate instruments. Avoid cutting sutures with them wherever possible.

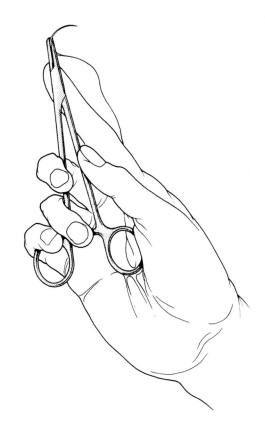

Figure 7.10   Controlling the needle-holder.

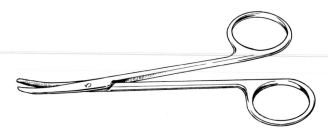

Figure 7.9   Positioning a needle in the needle-holder.

Figure 7.11   Dissecting scissors.

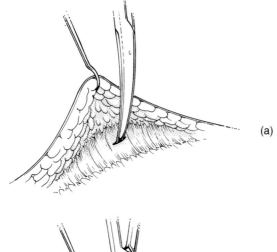

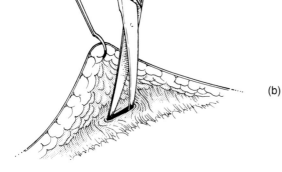

(a)

(b)

Figure 7.12 Blunt dissection. **(a)** Establishing a plane using dissecting scissors. **(b)** Dissecting a plane using dissecting scissors.

Suture scissors

Suture scissors have sharp points for precision cutting (Figure 7.13). They are more robust than dissecting scissors.

Scalpel

A scalpel handle and a selection of blades is best. For most minor surgery a number 15 blade is ideal (Figure 7.14). For shave excisions you will need a larger blade: a sterile safety razor blade is very satisfactory.

RETRACTORS

Skin hook

This is a tiny, very sharp hook on a handle (Figure 7.15).

It is essential for fine work. Position the hook in the subcutaneous tissue, deep to the wound edge itself, so that your assistant can use it to retract the wound edges without causing any damage.

Catspaw retractor

This retractor has two different ends (Figure 7.16).

The catspaw end is the most useful for minor skin surgery, when it may be used to retract the edge of the wound without damaging it.

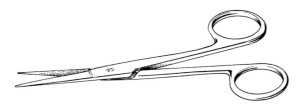

Figure 7.13 Suture scissors.

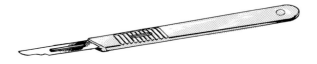

Figure 7.14 Scalpel handle with size 15 blade.

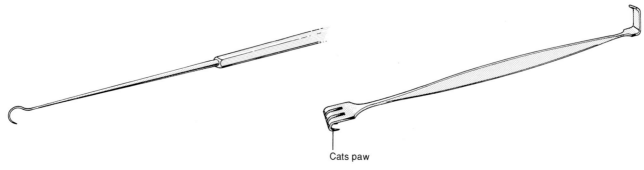

Cats paw

Figure 7.15 Skin hook.

Figure 7.16 Catspaw retractor.

SUTURES

SUTURE MATERIAL

There is a bewildering array of sutures available. As with instruments, get to know a small selection well. Choose one or two from each category and experiment with them.

Non-absorbable sutures are used for closing most skin wounds. They remain in tissue indefinitely and so have to be removed. Absorbable ones are eventually broken down at different rates depending on the type of suture. Both types may be made either from biological or synthetic material. They may consist of a single strand (**monofilament**), or many fine strands braided together (**multifilament**).

Non-absorbable sutures

Most doctors are familiar with black silk, which is a braided multifilament. Since it is very easy to tie, it is the suture that most people learn to use first. Its disadvantage is that it tends to excite a tissue reaction, resulting in an unsightly scar. Synthetic non-absorbable sutures are superior alternatives, and you could now be criticized for using a suture known to be prone to poor results.

We therefore recommend strongly that you do not use silk but the synthetic alternatives instead. An exception to this is wounds in the hair-bearing area of the scalp, where silk can be perfectly satisfactory.

There is a large range of man-made non-absorbable sutures, mostly known by their trade names – Prolene, Ethilon, etc. The most useful are the various types of monofilament suture, which consist of a single strand of smooth, nylon-like material. This glides smoothly through the tissue, is inert and excites virtually no tissue reaction. These sutures are excellent for most uses, including subcuticular closures. Their disadvantage is that they are more difficult to tie. Because they are less pliable than silk they tend to come undone. It is worth learning to use them, as they produce excellent results.

Absorbable sutures

These are used for suturing deeper layers and for tying blood vessels. In minor skin surgery this is seldom needed.

Catgut, made from sheep or cow intestine, is a monofilament, and may be plain or chromic. Plain catgut is untreated and loses its strength after 7–10

days. Chromic catgut has been treated with a solution of chromic salt so that it keeps its tensile strength for up to 28 days. Both kinds can produce a marked tissue reaction.

Polyglactin (Vicryl) and polyglycolic acid (Dexon) are multifilament sutures. They last much longer than catgut and produce little in the way of tissue reaction. In minor skin surgery their main use is for subcuticular stitches, where they have the advantage that they do not need to be removed. They can also be used if a deep suture is required for haemostasis.

SUTURE SIZES

There are two systems for describing the thickness of a suture: metric and traditional.

Metric

The number of the suture is equivalent to its diameter in tenths of a millimetre. A number 2 suture, for example, is 0.2 mm in diameter.

Traditional

Although less rational than the metric, the traditional system is still widely used. Suture thickness is expressed by an appropriate number of zeroes, e.g. 3/0, 4/0, 5/0 etc. The larger the number of zeroes, the finer the gauge of the suture. For the procedures described in this book, 3/0 is the thickest and 6/0 the finest suture that you will need.

SUMMARY OF RECOMMENDED SUTURES

- Prolene or Ethilon monofilament 1.5 metric (4/0) for interrupted skin sutures in most sites.
- Prolene or Ethilon monofilament 2 metric (3/0) for non-absorbable subcuticular closures; this can also be used for interrupted sutures on the back.
- Vicryl 2 metric (3/0) for absorbable subcuticular closures; this can also be used as a deep haemostatic suture.
- Prolene or Ethilon monofilament 0.7 metric (6/0) for fine facial work and in children.

NEEDLES

The most widely used type of needle is the 'atraumatic'. This description dates back to the days when most needles had an eye through which to thread the suture. As the needle passed through tissue it first made a hole the diameter of the needle, then a bigger hole because of the loop of suture – it was therefore traumatic (Figure 7.17).

Modern needles do not have eyes. The suture is **swaged** directly into a channel or hole in the butt end of the needle (Figure 7.18). The suture follows the needle causing no further damage, hence 'atraumatic' (Figure 7.19).

Most needles are curved, although the size of the needle and its degree of curvature can vary (Figure 7.20). Occasionally a straight needle can be useful,

especially for suturing long straight skin wounds with a subcuticular stitch, but in minor surgery such needles are usually unnecessary.

The most important distinctive feature is the shape of the point, defined as the area between the extreme tip of the needle and the maximum cross section of the body. This may not be easy to see, especially if the needle is very small, but there is always a description on the packet with a symbol for quick identification (Figure 7.21).

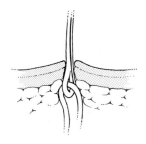

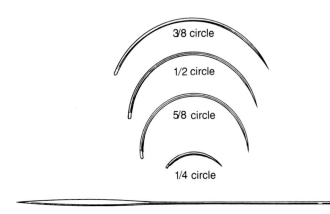

Figure 7.18 A swaged atraumatic needle.

Figure 7.17 Traumatic needle.

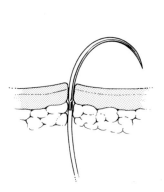

Figure 7.19 A swaged atraumatic needle emerging from the skin.

3/8 circle

1/2 circle

5/8 circle

1/4 circle

Figure 7.20 Curvatures of needle bodies.

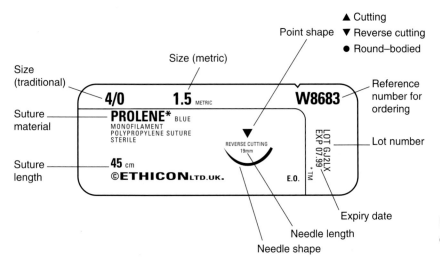

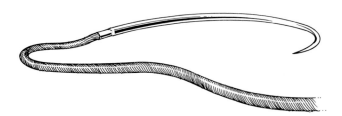

Point shape

▲ Cutting
▼ Reverse cutting
● Round–bodied

Size (traditional)

Size (metric)

4/0   **1.5** METRIC   **W8683**

Suture material

PROLENE* BLUE
MONOFILAMENT
POLYPROPYLENE SUTURE
STERILE

REVERSE CUTTING
19mm

LOT GJ2LX
EXP 07.99
* TM

Suture length

45 cm

©**ETHICON**LTD.UK.

E.O.

Reference number for ordering

Lot number

Expiry date

Needle length

Needle shape

Figure 7.21 Information provided on a suture pack.

CUTTING NEEDLES

Cutting needles have a triangular cross-section. There is a blade on each edge of the triangle so that the needle acts like three scalpels slicing through tissue. This is very effective for cutting skin, fascia and other tough tissue, but can cause tissue damage, especially in deeper parts of the body.

Conventional cutting needles

The apex of the triangle of edges is in the inner, concave curvature of the needle (Figure 7.22(a)). This makes it easier to pick up tissue.

Reverse cutting needles

In the reverse cutting needle, the apex of the triangle is on the outer, convex aspect (Figure 7.22(b)). It is said to have the advantage of reducing the likelihood of the needle cutting out to the edge of the incision.

In practice, either sort of cutting needle may be used.

ROUND-BODIED NEEDLES

Round-bodied needles are conical with a circular cross-section (Figure 7.22(c)). They are used for going through friable tissue. Its conical shape allows a round-bodied needle to push its way through mobile fibrous tissue, finding the path of least resistance. It behaves like someone shouldering his way through a crowd. However, if you try to force it through tough tissues such as skin or fascia it will easily bend or snap. Use a round-bodied needle to insert sutures deep in a wound – an unusual occurrence in minor surgery.

SUTURING

Principles

The cosmetic effect of a scar depends on the site of the wound and how well it heals.

SITE

A perfectly healed wound results in a thin linear scar. If the incision has been placed correctly and coincides with natural skin creases the scar will not be too noticeable. If it crosses the skin creases, however, it will be conspicuous and perhaps uncomfortable.

HEALING

Even a perfectly placed incision can result in an ugly scar if the wound becomes infected or breaks down. Blood supply to the edge of the wound is crucial. As soon as the wound edges come together healing by first intention begins. Coagulum binds the edges together, then fibroblasts move in and begin to unite them. This process is impaired if the blood supply is reduced, which happens if the wound is under tension or if its edges have been damaged by rough handling.

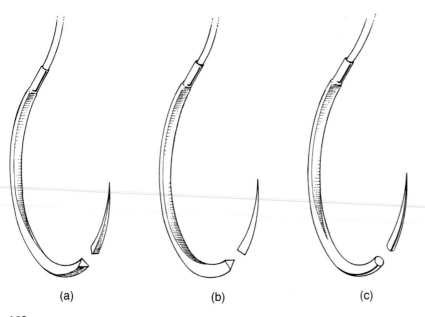

Figure 7.22
(a) Conventional cutting needle.
(b) Reverse cutting needle.
(c) Round-bodied needle.

(a)   (b)   (c)

Wound tension and trauma can be minimized in several ways.

- Careful attention to atraumatic technique, especially when handling the wound and putting in sutures, is vital. While you are suturing, an assistant can stabilize the wound by exerting gentle traction on a skin hook placed at each end.
- Undermining the edges of the wound using dissecting scissors or a scalpel with its blade held flat allows you to free the edge of the wound from the deep tissue (Figure 7.23). This technique is especially useful on the face. Take great care not to undermine too far, as you may make matters worse by reducing the blood supply.
- Occasionally you may need to appose the deeper parts of the wound with an absorbable suture so that the skin edges come together easily. Deep sutures will rarely be necessary during the procedures described but they may be helpful when removing large lesions.

TIGHTNESS

Wound edges swell quickly and continue swelling over the first 24 hours or so. If sutures are inserted too tightly they are likely to tighten further as the wound swells. This may cause ischaemia and necrosis with breakdown of the wound. You should allow for this inevitable swelling by putting sutures

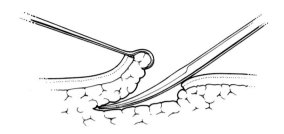

Figure 7.23 Undermining.

in loosely so that they lie comfortably without puckering the skin or biting into it. If the wound is properly designed there should be no need to haul protesting edges together.

Suturing technique

A curved needle travelling along a curved path will cause no more trauma than a straight needle travelling straight. A curved needle being forced straight, however, may do a lot of harm.

A curved needle follows the line of its curvature as it goes through tissue. Therefore consider the needle as describing a circle that begins before the needle touches the skin and continues after leaving it (Figure 7.24(a)–(d)). It is the principle of the golf swing.

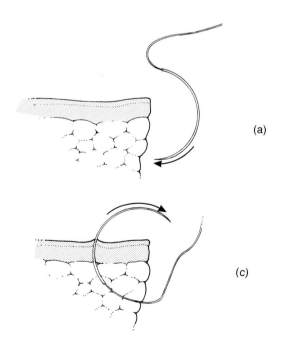

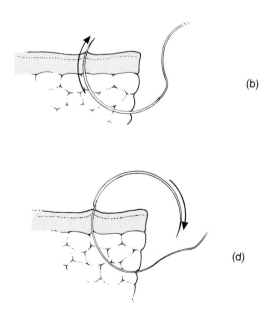

Figure 7.24(a)–(d) Using a curved needle correctly.

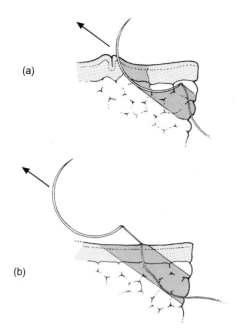

Figure 7.25(a) and (b) Using a curved needle incorrectly.

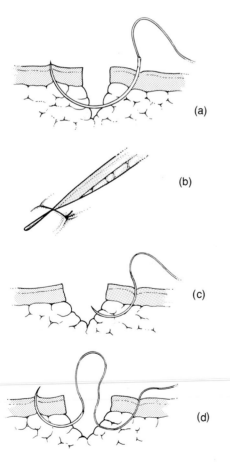

Figure 7.26(a)–(d) Simple interrupted sutures.

If you try to pull the needle out straight you will either damage the wound, if the needle is a strong one (Figure 7.25(a)), or buckle the needle, if it is not (Figure 7.25(b)).

INTERRUPTED SUTURES

Simple

The best all-purpose suture is the simple interrupted (Figure 7.26(a), (b)).

Equal bites of tissue are taken on each side of the wound. The suture crosses the wound and the knot is placed to one side.

For a short wound with sides of equal length it is best to start suturing at one end and go to the other. If the wound is long or the sides are unequal, use 'progressive halving' (p. 109).

Make sure that you take a large enough bite with the needle on each side. If the suture is too close to the edge of the wound it will produce an unsatisfactory result. Imagine the suture passing right under the wound and up at the other side. A useful rule of thumb is to make the distance between sutures about the same as the distance between the wound edge and the point at which the needle enters or leaves the skin.

If you are using a small needle do not try to bridge the whole wound, but bring the needle out halfway before piercing the other side (Figure 7.26(c), (d)).

It is important to **evert** the edges of the wound by taking a large bite of the deeper part of the tissue (Figure 7.27).

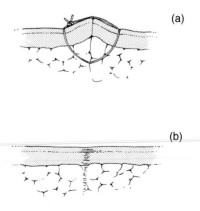

Figure 7.27 Everting the wound – correct technique. **(a)** Immediately after suturing. **(b)** Final result.

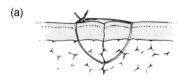

(a)

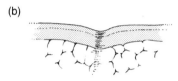

(b)

Figure 7.28 Failing to evert the wound – incorrect technique. **(a)** Immediately after suturing. **(b)** Final result.

If the wound edges are **inverted** the resulting scar will be depressed and ugly (Figure 7.28). Moving the knot can be a useful way of making fine adjustments to the edges.

Mattress

There is no place for mattress sutures in the type of surgery described here.

CONTINUOUS SUTURE

The continuous subcuticular stitch is extremely useful. Provided it is inserted without tension it can produce a scar that is almost invisible. This suture lies in a different plane from most others. It snakes to and fro **parallel** to the surface of the skin rather than at right angles to it. For this reason it does not have the strength to overcome tension in the wound.

Start a short distance from one end of the wound, guiding the needle point through the skin and coming out in the subcuticular plane. Grasp the needle-free end of the suture with artery forceps to stop it pulling through. Then take a series of looping bites in the subcuticular layer. Each new bite should start exactly opposite the point where the previous bite came out (Figure 7.29(a)).

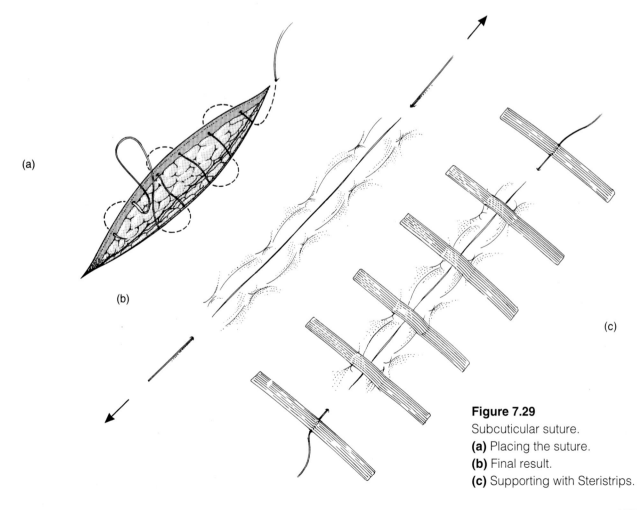

(a)

(b)

(c)

Figure 7.29
Subcuticular suture.
(a) Placing the suture.
(b) Final result.
(c) Supporting with Steristrips.

The whole suture can be inserted loosely and drawn up at the end. This allows you to see what you are doing all the time. When you reach the end of the wound, bring the needle out through the skin as you did at the beginning (Figure 7.29(b)).

The technique depends on friction to hold the wound edges together. It does not work satisfactorily if too fine a suture is used. 3/0 is recommended for most wounds. We favour a synthetic non-absorbable suture. To remove it, simply grasp one end and pull steadily. Do not make any knots in the suture or it will be impossible to remove. The ends are most easily secured using Steristrips, which may also be used to close any gaps in the wound and to give it additional support (Figure 7.29(c)). The whole wound can then be buttressed with flesh-coloured adhesive tape.

An alternative is to use a synthetic absorbable suture such as Dexon or Vicryl, in which case, in theory, the suture does not need to be removed. In practice, however, patients often complain of persistent discomfort because the suture takes a long time to disappear.

Tying knots

For any surgery it is essential to know how to tie a reliable knot. The reef knot is ideal for most purposes. A reef knot is symmetrical, lies flat and gets tighter when the ends are pulled (Figure 7.30(a)). A granny knot, on the other hand, is asymmetrical and tends to come undone (Figure 7.30(b)).

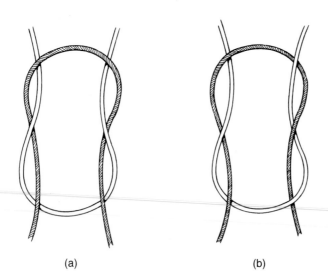

(a)   (b)

Figure 7.30   (a) Reef knot.   **(b)** Granny knot.

If the suture material is fine it is impossible to see the type of knot you have made. You must therefore be confident that you have tied the knot in such a way that you **know** it is safe. It is worth slowly analysing how you tie a knot. With practice it will soon become second nature.

A needle-holder should be used for tying sutures since it allows you to place the sutures precisely and to control the tightness of the knot. It is preferable to learn to use a needle-holder properly than to waste time on one-handed tying techniques, which in any case waste suture material.

Having inserted a suture, grasp the needle in your non-dominant hand. Hold the needle-holder in your dominant hand to manipulate the other end of the suture.

TYING TECHNIQUE

A reef knot consists of two throws. For each throw loop one end of thread round the other like the first part of a shoelace bow. It does not matter which direction you start with. Having made the first throw pull the ends of the suture so that the throw stays flat as you tighten it (Figure 7.31(a), (b)).

The next throw must be in the other direction, so that by the time you have tied the second throw, the ends will also be pointing in the other direction. This is the direction in which you must pull to tighten the knot (Figure 7.31(c), (d)).

Thus each throw has two components – a direction of **throw** and a direction of **pull**. Each component must be changed as you tie the knot.

SPECIAL TECHNIQUES

Tying knots in silk is usually easy. Since silk has a high coefficient of friction the first throw tends to stay in position until you have tied the second.

Many people find that synthetic monofilament non-absorbable sutures such as Prolene are much more difficult to tie. The suture material seems to have a life of its own. The first throw starts to come undone before you have had a chance to make the second. The suture may not stay where you put it, particularly if there is the slightest traction from a gaping wound.

Using these sutures requires skill. It is a skill well worth learning, however, as the results are so much better than using silk. To prevent the first throw from unravelling 'lock' it temporarily, as follows (Figure 7.32).

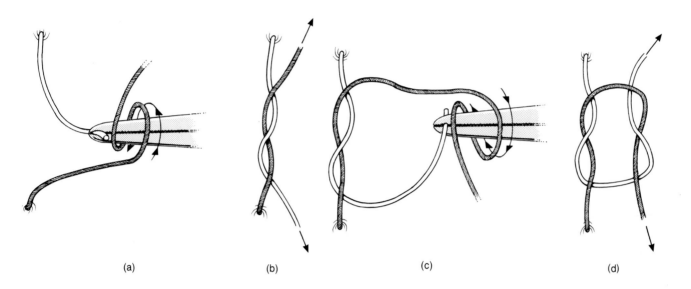

Figure 7.31 Tying a reef knot. **(a) and (b)** First throw; **(c) and (d)** Second throw.

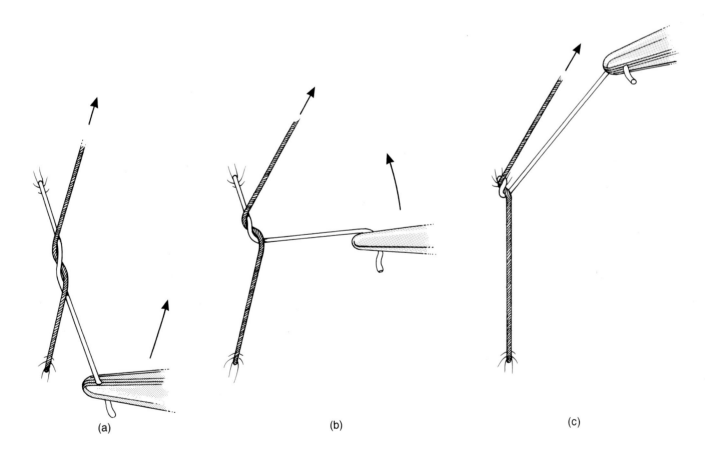

Figure 7.32(a)–(c) 'Locking' the first throw.

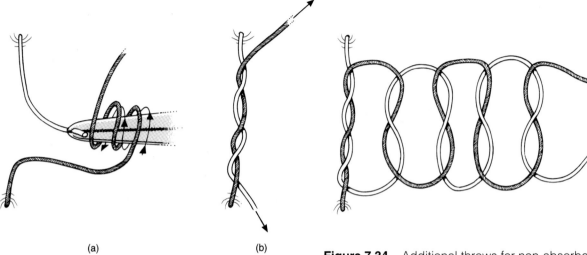

(a)   (b)

Figure 7.33(a) and (b)   Additional turn in first throw.

Figure 7.34   Additional throws for non-absorbable synthetic sutures.

Adjust the tension of the first throw until it is satisfactory, then continue pulling one end of the suture with your non-dominant hand, while moving the end in the needle-holder sharply in the same direction, tightening the throw. You can then make the second throw without difficulty (Figure 7.32).

Another method to increase the grip is to make a 'surgeon's knot', by putting an additional turn into the first throw (Figure 7.33).

Because synthetic monofilament non-absorbable sutures tend to slip it is important to put additional throws in the knot. Each throw makes a reef knot with the one before it and it is possible to build up a whole series of these into a composite knot (Figure 7.34). Five throws are usually sufficient. Remember that the direction of the throw and the pull must alternate.

TRAPS FOR THE UNWARY

If you do not change the direction of throw at each of the two stages you will make a granny knot (Figure 7.35).

If you change the direction of **throw** but not the direction of **pull** you will make a slip knot (Figure 7.36). This is surprisingly easy to do if you do not concentrate.

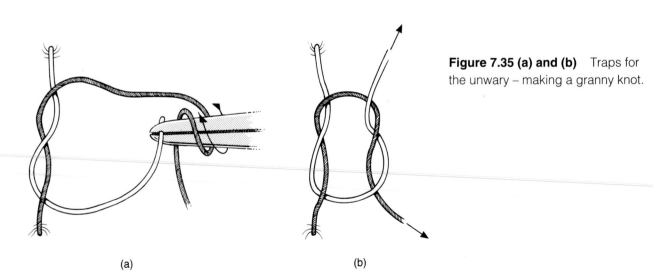

Figure 7.35 (a) and (b)   Traps for the unwary – making a granny knot.

(a)   (b)

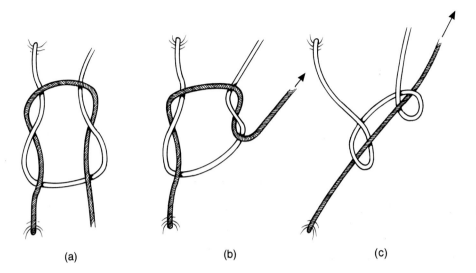

Figure 7.36 (a)–(c) Traps for the unwary – making a slip knot.

Wound problems

As the surgeon making the wound, you have control over most of the factors that affect healing. Nevertheless, you may sometimes misjudge the incision and produce a wound with unequal sides or a 'dog ear'.

PROGRESSIVE HALVING FOR UNEVEN LENGTHS

If you insert sutures proceeding from one end of the wound you may find an excess of tissue on the longer side when you reach the other end. This extra tissue is bunched up in one place, leading to an ugly 'dog ear' (Figure 7.37).

Progressive halving can be useful here. Find the midpoint of each side of the wound and insert your first suture (Figure 7.38(a)). Then insert sutures at the midpoint of each of the two resulting halves (Figure 7.38(b)). Continue this process along the whole wound. In this way the extra length of the longer side is distributed equally along the wound so that even fairly large discrepancies become unnoticeable (Figure 7.38(c)).

Progressive halving may also be helpful when the edges of a wound can only be brought together under tension. A loosely tied central suture can relieve the tension at the ends of the wound. Progressive halving will reduce this tension further.

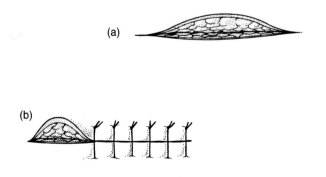

Figure 7.37 Uneven wound edges. **(a)** Uneven edges. **(b)** 'Dog ear'.

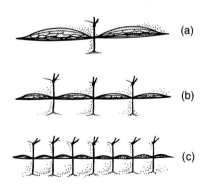

Figure 7.38(a)–(c) Progressive halving.

Finally you should remove the central suture and reinsert it.

A 'dog ear' is an unsightly bunching-up of skin at the end of a sutured wound. It may be easily dealt with as shown in Figure 7.39.

REMOVING SUTURES

The insertion of a suture makes a track through the skin which quickly becomes lined with fibroblasts. If sutures are left in too long, scars appear at the site of insertion and cause ugly cross-markings. It is therefore important to remove sutures as soon as possible. If you take them out too soon, however, the wound may gape. A general guide is as follows:

- **most sutures:** remove after 7–10 days;
- **face:** remove in 5 days at the most; support the wound with Steristrips after removing sutures;
- **difficult areas (e.g. back, leg, foot):** remove after 14 days or longer; again, you may wish to support the wound with Steristrips after removing sutures.

Removing sutures is an important part of the operation often delegated to the practice nurse. It must be done gently with fine instruments in a good light. You should make sure that anyone who removes sutures has the necessary skills.

PROCEDURES

Excising a lesion

First confirm with the patient which lesion you are going to excise. Mark the lesion with a pen, especially if it is deep, or you may be unable to find it after infiltrating around it with local anaesthetic.

Always mark out the proposed incision on the skin before cutting anything. Any adjustments can easily be made at this stage before committing yourself to a scar by incising the skin. Bear in mind that when you cover the patient with sterile towels you will find it more difficult to get your bearings. A felt-tipped marker pen is satisfactory, provided it will not wash off immediately with antiseptic solution.

Even if your incision is elliptical the result will be a linear wound. Consider first where you want this line to lie and mark each end of it on the skin with a dot. Then draw the ellipse, making sure it encompasses the lesion adequately.

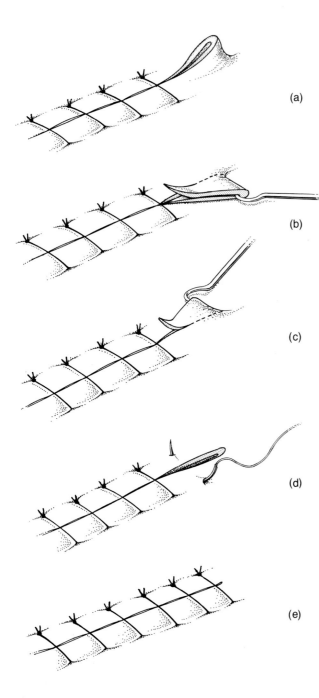

(a)

(b)

(c)

(d)

(e)

Figure 7.39 Technique for removing a 'dog ear'.
(a) The 'dog ear'. **(b)** Pull the 'dog ear' flat to one side using a skin hook and incise as shown. **(c)** Pull the 'dog ear' flat to the other side and make a second incision as shown to remove the redundant skin.
(d) and (e) Insert an additional suture.

If you cut through marked skin there is a possibility of embedding pigment particles and causing a tattoo. To avoid this, design your marked ellipse so that the incision will be just outside it (Figure 7.40). Then infiltrate with local anaesthetic and wait for it to take effect (p. 87–8).

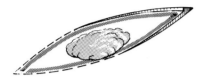

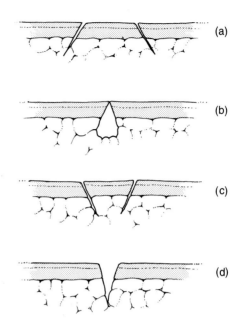

Figure 7.42(a)–(d) Making a vertical incision: incorrect technique using slanting incisions.

Figure 7.40 Marking and making an elliptical excision.

Ellipse excision

Once you are ready to start, make a bold incision through the full thickness of the skin. Avoid tentative scratching. Keep to the marks you have made and do not modify the incision when you start to cut. Make sure your scalpel is at right angles to the surface of the skin (Figure 7.41). The two wound edges should be vertical so that they come together neatly. A slanting incision produces a chamfered edge which may result in poor healing (Figure 7.42).

It is all too easy to allow the two sides of the incision to cross at the points (Figure 7.43(a)). This gives an ugly fishtail effect. To avoid this, first cut each point towards the centre then join each edge up in the middle (Figure 7.43(b)).

Having made the incision, ensure that it is deep enough. It is important to remove a margin of tissue around the lesion **in all directions**. Remove the specimen and put it in a specimen pot. Then make sure that the edges of the wound will come together without tension. If necessary some judicious undermining of the wound edges can be very helpful. Before closing the wound, ensure that haemostasis is satisfactory.

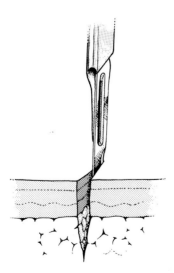

Figure 7.41 Making a vertical incision: correct technique.

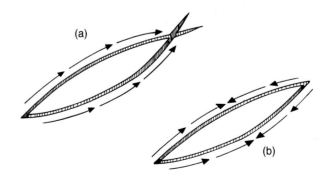

Figure 7.43 Making an ellipse incision.
(a) Incorrect technique showing fishtail effect at corner.
(b) Recommended technique.

Epidermoid cysts

As it grows, an epidermoid cyst pushes itself into the surrounding tissues. If it has not been infected there is a clear plane of cleavage around it and with careful dissection it can usually be removed complete. If there is a history of previous infection, however, the cyst may be firmly embedded in fibrous tissue, making the operation much more of a challenge.

A central punctum is usually identifiable in the skin overlying the cyst. The punctum is its only point of attachment to the skin and it should be excised using an elliptical incision.

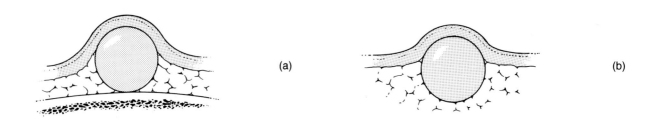

Figure 7.44   Enlargement of epidermoid cyst.   **(a)** Firm base leads to enlargement outwards.   **(b)** Soft base allows enlargement inwards.

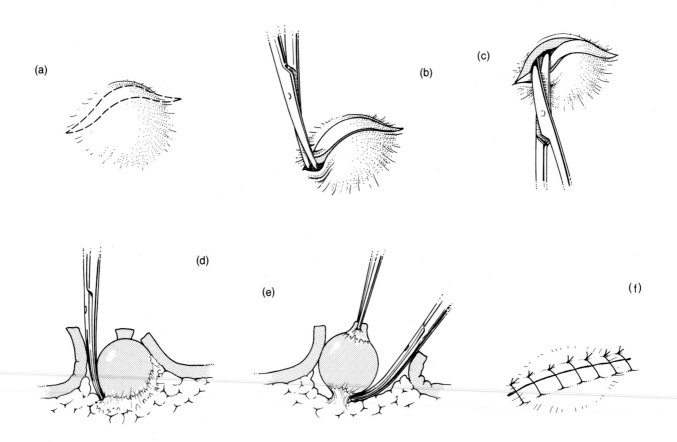

Figure 7.45(a)–(f)   Diagrammatic representation of removal of an epidermoid cyst.

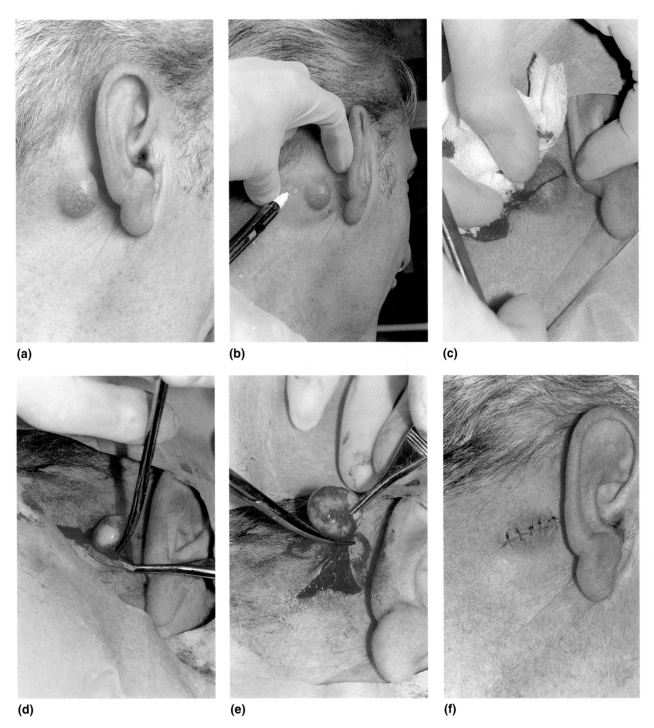

(a)   **(b)**   **(c)**

(d)   **(e)**   **(f)**

Figure 7.46   Removal of an epidermoid cyst.   **(a)** Epidermoid cyst behind the ear.   **(b)** Infiltrating with local anaesthetic.   **(c)** Making the first part of the ellipse over the cyst.   **(d)** Careful dissection around the cyst. **(e)** Intact cyst being removed.   **(f)** Wound closed with fine synthetic non-absorbable sutures.

The size of the ellipse depends on the size and site of the cyst. On the scalp, for example, it cannot enlarge downwards because of bone. It grows upwards instead, stretching the overlying skin (Figure 7.44(a)).

You should therefore remove a large ellipse so

that there is no redundant skin after removal of the cyst. Other cysts enlarge downwards, causing only slight stretching of the skin (Figure 7.44(b)). Even if the cyst is large you will only need a small ellipse. If you make the ellipse too large, skin closure will be difficult.

As you make the skin incision, be very careful not to cut into the cyst, which lies very close to the skin surface. Start dissecting at the edge of the incision, where the cyst is curving away from you. Here you can cut deeply without danger of puncturing the cyst. Once you have established the correct plane it is easy to develop it, using a combination of cutting and blunt dissection (Figures 7.45, 7.46).

It is not a disaster if the cyst bursts. However, to avoid recurrence you should try to remove the cyst wall complete. If the cyst bursts at the beginning of the procedure, an alternative technique is to pick up the deep wall with artery forceps and pull the cyst inside out.

In some circumstances this technique is to be preferred. After expressing the contents of the cyst via a small incision, reach in and grasp the wall with artery forceps, and dissect it free with small curved scissors. This is particularly suitable for small cysts on the face and can produce excellent results with minimal scarring.

Chapter 8

Practical skills: dermatological techniques

CURETTAGE

Curettage is a very useful technique that allows some benign lesions to be removed and sent for histological examination. Because it involves the removal of very superficial tissue it gives excellent cosmetic results in selected patients. In particular, it is the treatment of choice for basal cell papillomas (seborrhoeic keratoses).

During the procedure the curette either scrapes a surface lesion off the skin or hugs a deeper lesion, developing a plane of cleavage around it. The advantage of the technique is that it causes minimal scarring. The disadvantage is that, unlike excision, it does not allow you to remove a margin of normal tissue. It is therefore unsuitable for dealing with malignant lesions unless you have special experience.

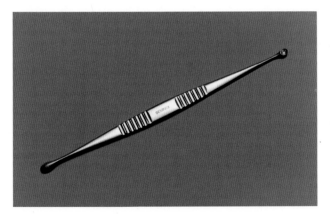

Figure 8.1 Volkmann double-ended curette.

Curettage combined with electrocautery is used by many dermatologists, for example in the treatment of basal cell carcinomas, but precise details of the technique are very important. We recommend that you use the curette only if you are confident that the lesion is benign.

TECHNIQUE

A curette is simply a long handled sharpened spoon. It may be double-ended with one larger and one smaller spoon (Figure 8.1).

The edges of the curette are only slightly sharpened so that it is impossible to cut through normal intact skin. However, it is possible to develop a plane of cleavage around a lesion and to separate it from the surrounding tissue.

The instrument may be used in two ways. In the first the curette is held flat to scrape the lesion off the surface of the skin. In the second it digs more deeply to scoop the lesion out.

Scraping

This is the ideal technique for removing basal cell papillomas. These are only lightly attached to the skin, as if by a thin layer of glue, and may be easily removed by firm scraping using a sideways movement of the curette (Figure 8.2).

The curettings obtained, even though fragmented, should be sent for histological examination.

This procedure leaves a raw area oozing tiny spots of blood. The bleeding may be stopped by direct pressure, by electrocautery or by application

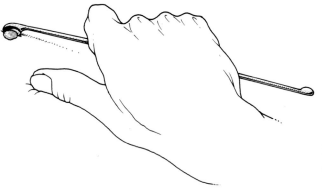

Figure 8.2 Using the curette to scrape off a basal cell papilloma.

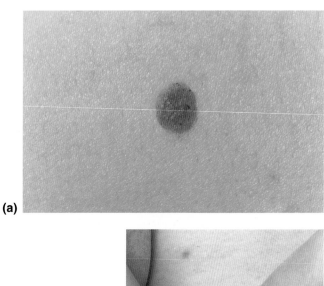

(a)

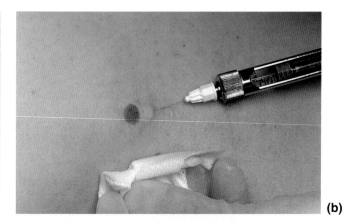

(b)

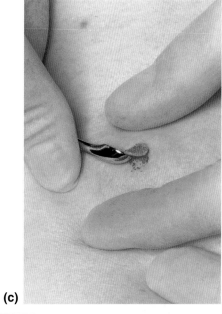

(c)

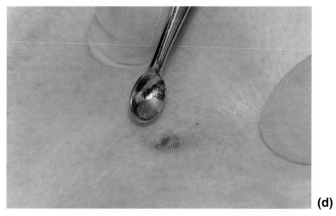

(d)

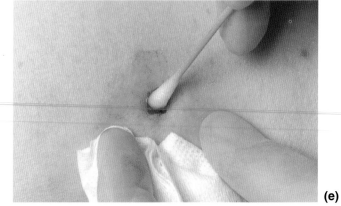

(e)

Figure 8.3 Curettage of basal cell papilloma.
(a) Basal cell papilloma on trunk. **(b)** Infiltrating with local anaesthetic. **(c)** Scraping the lesion firmly with the curette. **(d)** Resulting wound (the lesion is in the curette). **(e)** Securing haemostasis with aluminium chloride solution on a cotton bud.

of aluminium chloride solution (25% aluminium chloride in 70% isopropyl alcohol) on a cotton bud. After a few days this superficial wound will have healed completely leaving virtually no sign (Figure 8.3).

Ellipse excision of a basal cell papilloma is inappropriate as it leaves an unnecessary scar.

Scooping

This alternative technique is used for pyogenic granulomas. The curette is held at right angles to the surface at the junction of the lesion and the normal skin. Using firm downward pressure, develop a plane of cleavage and scoop out the lesion from below (Figure 8.4). There may be profuse bleeding from the resulting hole, which should be dealt with by direct pressure or electrocautery.

ELECTROCAUTERY

In this technique a red-hot platinum wire is used to coagulate small blood vessels or to cut through tissue. It differs from diathermy in that it works solely by heat.

The main uses of electrocautery are:
- to remove or treat lesions, e.g. skin tags, spider naevi;
- to control bleeding, especially after curettage or shave excision;
- to destroy residual tissue, e.g. following curettage of basal cell carcinomas.

EQUIPMENT

Electrocautery machines consist of an electrical source and a range of platinum wire tips.

Electrocautery machines

Standard mains machines consist of a transformer, with a dial to control the current and therefore the temperature, together with a hand-held attachment into which the cautery tip is fitted (Figure 8.5).

The advantage of this type of machine is that it allows precise control of the temperature of the tip. However, it is rather cumbersome to use.

An alternative is a rechargeable machine which is not attached to the mains during use (Figure 8.6).

It has the advantage of being portable and more convenient. However, it is not possible to control the temperature, since the current is either on or off. Nevertheless, with experience the temperature of the

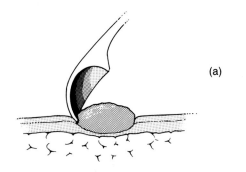
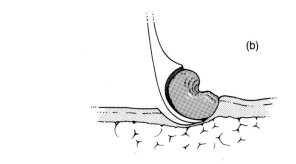

Figure 8.4 (a) and (b) Using the curette to scoop out a lesion.

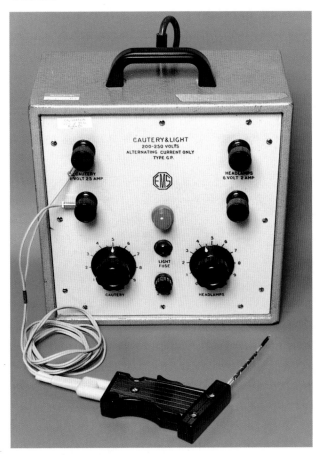

Figure 8.5 Mains-operated cautery machine.

wire can be varied by altering the time from heating to application. It is important to make sure that the batteries are adequately charged before each session. Disposable machines are expensive but may be convenient for occasional use.

Although dermatology departments usually have mains machines, the rechargeable cautery is excellent for general practice.

Electrocautery tips

There are three main types of electrocautery tip: the ball, the ring cutter (cutting tip) and the 'cold-point' burner. There are many variations of these basic designs. Each type is available in a long or short version. The short one is easier to use.

- **The coagulation ball tip**, which has a larger surface area than the cutting type, is used to stop bleeding without cutting through tissue (Figure 8.7(a)).
- **The ring cutting tip** is flat (Figure 8.7(b)). In addition to coagulating it cuts through tissue and is useful for removing skin tags.
- The **cold-point burner** has a fine central point with a heating wire wound round it (Figure 8.7(c)). The point can be positioned very precisely before it is heated. It is excellent for treating spider naevi. To confirm the diagnosis, use the end of a wire paper clip to press on the central feeding vessel, which should blanch. To treat the lesion, position the tip of the cold-point burner

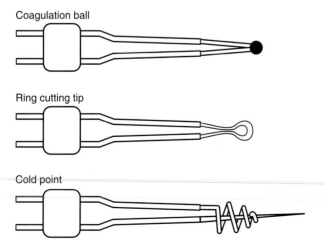
(a)

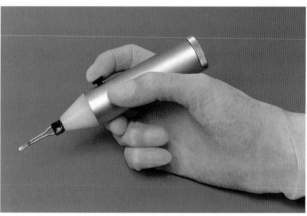
(b)

Figure 8.6 **(a)** Rechargeable electrocautery handle with charger and selection of tips. **(b)** Rechargeable electrocautery in use. (Reproduced by permission of Warecrest Ltd.)

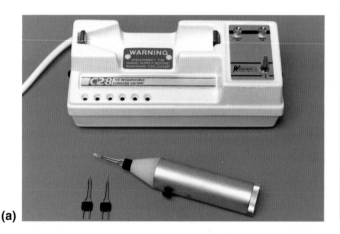

Figure 8.7 Electrocautery tips. **(a)** Ball tip. **(b)** Ring cutting tip. **(c)** Cold-point tip.

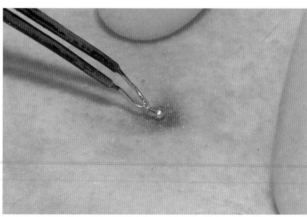

Figure 8.8 Using the electrocautery ball for haemostasis.

precisely in the centre of the vessel, then heat it for about 1 second. There is no need for local anaesthetic.

TECHNIQUE

The main use of the electocautery is haemostasis (Figure 8.8).

In general the best temperature is when the wire is a dull red colour. If the wire is too hot it cuts through tissue without coagulating; if it is not hot enough it sticks to the tissues.

It is important to remember that the heat produced by the electrocautery destroys tissue more widely than you can see. Consequently, if a histological specimen is required you should take a biopsy before using electocautery.

Never use spirit-based skin-cleaning solutions with electrocautery, since these may ignite and burn the patient.

DIATHERMY

Diathermy is another technique used to damage tissue in a controlled way. It depends on electricity rather than just heat to produce its effects. Diathermy machines produce a low current at high voltage and very high frequency.

The standard hospital operating theatre diathermy is **bipolar**. This means it has two electrodes: a large one in the form of a pad, usually attached to the patient's thigh, and a smaller one used by the surgeon to cut or coagulate tissue.

Unipolar diathermy uses only one electrode. The most widely used machine is the Birtcher Hyfrecator. It may be used in three ways:

- to **coagulate** tissue in a similar way to the electrocautery;
- to **fulgurate** tissue using the stream of sparks produced when it is held just above the lesion;
- to **desiccate** tissue by causing drying in a small area around the point of the Hyfrecator needle.

Although diathermy may be used in minor surgery the expense of the machine is not generally justified.

SHAVE EXCISION

Shave excision involves slicing off a lesion with a flat blade. It is a highly effective treatment for compound naevi, the fleshy lesions that often occur on the face, especially the cheek and lip. The attachment and depth of these lesions means that they should not be curetted. The technique produces an excellent cosmetic result, avoiding the need for sutures, and deserves to be more widely used than it is.

Because shave excision does not always remove the lesion completely, the histopathologist will be unable to report on the depth or the completeness of the excision. **The technique should therefore only be used if you are confident that the lesion is benign**.

You should warn patients in advance that they will be left with a hole which can look rather alarming. However, you can reassure them that this will heal rapidly and that the eventual results are usually excellent. Remember that repigmentation can take place, that the lesion may recur and that any hairs previously present in the lesion may grow back again.

TECHNIQUE

After infiltrating with local anaesthetic grasp the lesion with toothed forceps and draw it upwards slightly. Then hold a scalpel blade (11 or 15) or a

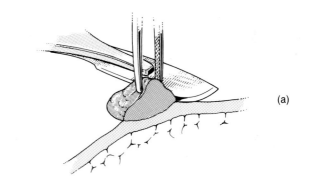

(a)

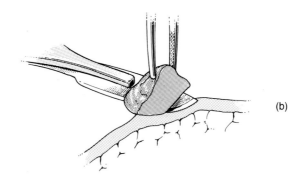

(b)

Figure 8.9(a) and (b) Shave excision.

sterile razor blade horizontally and slice off the lesion with a steady to and fro motion (Figures 8.9, 8.10).

Make the incision in such a way that the lesion is cut off flush with the skin, or even slightly deeper. A residual rim of lesion standing proud produces a conspicuous raised scar which casts a shadow. A flat or slightly concave scar, on the other hand, may be easily concealed with make-up.

Bleeding can usually be controlled by pressure or aluminium chloride (p. 115–16). An alternative is to use the ball end of the electrocautery. If you are using the electocautery near the nose remember to warn patients of the smell of singeing flesh. Reassure them that the black charred spot they will see in the mirror will heal quickly.

SNIP EXCISION

This is a quick, easy way to remove skin tags which are common on the neck, in the flexures and around the eyes.

SMALL TAGS

If the tags are very small a local anaesthetic is unnecessary: the injection itself would be more painful than cutting the tags. The tag is held firmly in a pair of forceps and snipped off at the base with a pair of sharp scissors. Haemostasis is not usually a problem. Patients can be shown how to perform the procedure themselves if small tags recur.

LARGER TAGS

For removal of larger skin tags local anaesthetic should be used. Again the tag is held firmly in the forceps and cut off at the base with scissors. Larger skin tags have a better developed blood supply and so cautery of the base, either with electrocautery or aluminium chloride, may be required for haemostasis. Alternatively the electrocautery cutting tip (ring cutter) can be used.

CRYOTHERAPY

Background

Cryotherapy is the therapeutic use of cold to destroy tissue. It works by producing ice crystals in the intracellular and extracellular fluids. Freezing followed by thawing causes intracellular damage which leads to tissue necrosis. Liquid nitrogen is the most widely used agent and by far the best. Other agents such as carbon dioxide snow are now of historical interest only.

Liquid nitrogen has a boiling point of –196°C. It is non-toxic and non-inflammable but can nevertheless be dangerous and should be treated with great respect. It can be used in several ways to apply cold with precision and control.

Cryotherapy is simple to perform and does not usually require local anaesthesia. This apparent simplicity can be deceptive, however, and it is essential to master the details of the technique in order to use it successfully. Freezing for too short a time is

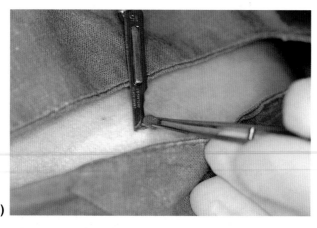
(a)

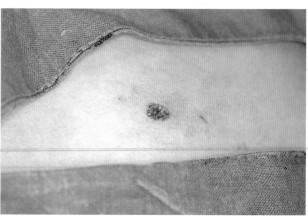
(b)

Figure 8.10 Shave excision. **(a)** Slicing through the base of the lesion. **(b)** Wound following shave excision and cautery.

ineffective, while freezing for too long can cause serious damage to surrounding tissue.

A major disadvantage is that cryotherapy does not **remove** tissue, so you cannot confirm the diagnosis histologically. This means that you must be absolutely certain of the diagnosis before considering this technique.

The ease and apparent harmlessness of the technique can make it seem attractive, and cryotherapy has been advocated for treating a tremendous range of lesions, including some skin malignancies. This is a dangerous practice. Unless you have special experience in this field it is safest to confine your use of cryotherapy to treating viral warts, solar keratoses and basal cell papillomas.

> **Golden rule:** *never embark on treatment with cryotherapy unless you are confident of the diagnosis and sure that it is appropriate treatment.*

INDICATIONS

Viral warts

Treating viral warts is the main indication for cryotherapy in general practice. However this does not mean that all viral warts require such treatment. Most warts in healthy individuals resolve spontaneously. If your patients think that you are offering an easy treatment for warts your practice will be inundated with requests for it. Insist that patients try a prolonged course of a topical anti-wart preparation before you consider cryotherapy (see p. 18). Remember too that cryotherapy is painful and should be avoided in children.

Solar keratoses

Cryotherapy is the treatment of choice for solar keratoses, **provided that the diagnosis is not in doubt**. See Chapter 1 for further information about the management of solar keratoses.

Basal cell papillomas

Cryotherapy can be used for basal cell papillomas provided that the diagnosis is not in doubt. See Chapter 1 for further information about management of basal cell papillomas.

EQUIPMENT

Liquid nitrogen

Liquid nitrogen may be bought in bulk and stored in a large Dewar flask where it will last for up to 3 months. In general practice, however, it is usually more convenient to arrange with the local hospital to supply small amounts when needed. Because the boiling point of liquid nitrogen is so low it evaporates continuously and needs to be kept in a specially designed insulated container. A litre of liquid nitrogen in such a container will last for about a day. You should wear gloves and goggles when transferring liquid nitrogen from one container to another.

You must also have a special vented flask to transport liquid nitrogen. You should ensure that this is kept upright at all times and that the vent is clear. If you are driving with the flask in the car you should ensure that the vehicle is well ventilated. **An ordinary domestic Thermos flask is unsuitable for transporting liquid nitrogen and can be dangerous.**

Cryospray (Figure 8.11)

Cryospray instruments consist of a double-insulated metal flask with a screw top. This is fitted with a

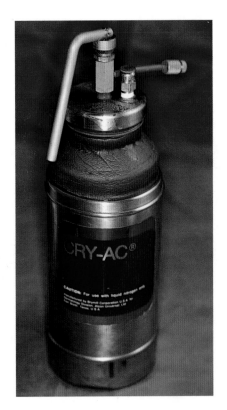

Figure 8.11 Cryospray with nozzles.

trigger device and a choice of metal nozzles with different-sized apertures. This allows the controlled delivery of a fine spray of liquid nitrogen, that can be aimed precisely.

The cryospray avoids any risk of contamination since the instrument does not touch the patient's skin. It is easy to use and a short period of practice using simulated tissue or an orange will enable you to master the technique.

TECHNIQUE

Cotton bud

Cotton buds are dipped into a flask of liquid nitrogen and applied to the lesion. This is the simplest technique and is widely used, but it is not as effective as the cryospray.

Commercially available cotton buds are too loosely packed to be satisfactory. Make your own by twisting a wisp of cotton wool around the end of an orange stick. Although freezing destroys wart-infected tissue the virus itself is not destroyed by the procedure. Never dip a used cotton bud into the liquid nitrogen flask or you may cause cross-infection.

Cryospray

Select a suitable nozzle size and direct a fine jet of liquid nitrogen on to the lesion from a distance of about 1 cm. After a short time the lesion will freeze and turn white (Figure 8.12).

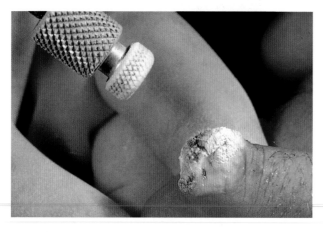

Figure 8.12 Treating a viral wart with liquid nitrogen. (Reproduced with permission from Brown, J.S. (1992) *Minor Surgery: A text and atlas*, 2nd edn, Chapman & Hall, London.)

Start counting the freeze time from this point and continue spraying for between 5 and 10 seconds. Time this carefully and record the freeze time in the procedure notes.

Recommended freeze times

- **Common digital or plantar warts:** 10 seconds
- **Solar keratoses:** 5 seconds
- **Basal cell papillomas:** 5 seconds; large raised basal cell papillomas may need longer.

Freeze–thaw cycles

There is evidence that two freeze–thaw cycles are more efficient than a single application. Treat the lesion with liquid nitrogen until it goes white, then stop the treatment and allow the area to return to its normal colour before repeating the cycle.

COMPLICATIONS

Cryotherapy is safe if used correctly, but because it appears so simple it is easy to overlook its dangers. Applying it for too long can cause devastating results. A maximum freeze time of 10 seconds is recommended for most lesions.

Pain and blistering

Although cryotherapy itself does not require local anaesthesia, it can cause severe pain after the procedure. It is most important to explain to the patient the likely effects of treatment, which may be described as a 'freeze burn'. An information leaflet should be supplied. Explain that pain, inflammation, redness and blister formation are to be expected over the next few days. The blister, which is often haem-orrhagic, can be punctured to make it more comfortable. It is probably not necessary to induce blister formation in order to treat viral warts. There are no hard and fast rules about application of dressings to areas treated with cryotherapy. Advise patients to dress the lesion as they would a similar wound elsewhere on the body.

Scarring

Scarring may occur if freeze times are prolonged. The nail bed is particularly liable to damage when resistant periungual warts are being treated. This can cause distortion of the nail.

Nerve damage

Paraesthesia and anaesthesia can result from prolonged freezing near peripheral nerves. This is often temporary but may be permanent.

Depigmentation

Changes in pigmentation after cryotherapy are an important complication. Temporary postinflammatory hypopigmentation is common, but hyperpigmentation may also occur. Sometimes these changes may be permanent. Dark-skinned people are at particular risk and the possibility of pigment changes should always be explained before undertaking the procedure.

Tendon rupture

Tendon rupture has been reported after prolonged treatment of warts on the hands. The extensor tendons in particular lie perilously close to the skin. Take particular care when treating warts on the sides of the fingers.

OUTCOME

Viral warts

Most warts require more than one treatment. The cure rate is related to the number of treatments rather than the interval between them. More rapid cure will be achieved by shortening the time between treatments to weekly or fortnightly. When treating warts more frequently, avoid retreating a wart that is still blistered.

Cryotherapy does not cure all viral warts. Studies have shown that many warts that fail to resolve spontaneously within 3 months or fail to respond to wart paints also fail to respond to cryotherapy. After 12 treatments cure rates are around 40–50%. Repeated freezing of unresponsive warts is rarely of value.

Combination therapy using a topical salicylic acid preparation (wart paint) between cryotherapy treatments has been shown to be more effective than cryotherapy alone. However, in the first few days after cryotherapy the site may be too sore to apply wart paint. The patient should be advised to restart application of the wart paint as soon as the inflammatory response from cryotherapy has settled.

Solar keratoses and basal cell papillomas

Similar principles apply to treating solar keratoses and basal cell papillomas. A freeze time of 5 seconds is recommended and more than one treatment is often necessary. Large or raised basal cell papillomas may need up to 10 seconds. The interval between treatments should be 3–4 weeks. If the lesion is on the face ensure that the nuisance of post-treatment inflammation and blistering will not happen at a socially inconvenient time.

See Chapter 1 for alternative treatments for these conditions.

Chapter 9
Skills training

Some of the procedures referred to in this book may be unfamiliar to you. Others may have been familiar in the past, but not now. In either case you will need practical experience of particular skills.

Naturally you should be fully competent and feel confident before operating on a patient. Before carrying out a new procedure it is essential to gain experience under the guidance of an experienced colleague. There is a learning curve for all procedures and you can never step on to a learning curve at the top.

USE OF SIMULATED TISSUE

When you are learning a new technique it can be very helpful to practise on an artificial substitute. Recent advances have led to the development of sophisticated models of particular parts of the body specially designed for training.

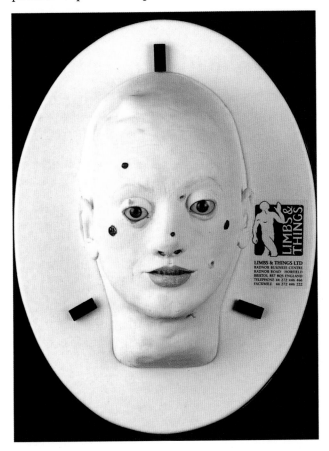

Figure 9.1   Simulated face. (Reproduced by permission of Limbs & Things Ltd, Bristol.)

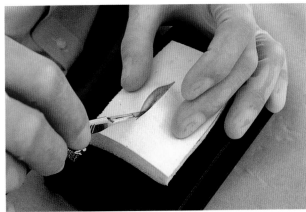

Figure 9.2   Jig with skin pad for practising surgical techniques.

Some are highly realistic models (Figure 9.1). In addition, pads of 'tissue' may be used for practising certain techniques, e.g. excising lesions, suturing wounds, curettage and electrocautery (Figure 9.2).

Using these models doctors can practise under non-stressful conditions until they have mastered the necessary skills for operating on patients. Models are useful for developing basic skills, for keeping up to date with new techniques, and for retaining infrequently used skills.

Epilogue

Much of this book has attempted to remove any uncertainty you may have about the diagnosis of skin lesions and enable you to make rational decisions about appropriate management.

We have emphasized the many pitfalls, and it is easy to get the impression that minor surgery is more trouble than it is worth. But this is not the case at all. On the contrary, managing patients with skin lesions is a fundamental part of general practice. People are increasingly consulting their family doctors about skin lesions, especially as publicity campaigns raise awareness of skin cancer, particularly malignant melanoma.

Much of the uneasiness that many doctors feel in this area stems from a lack of confidence in diagnosis. However, dermatology need not be an intimidating subject. Much of it depends on pattern recognition and once you have seen the common lesions you will know them again. Even the spectre of misdiagnosing a malignant melanoma loses much of its terror when you realize that by following simple management guidelines you will be able to practise safe medicine.

You will be able to treat many lesions yourself, and provided you are competent this makes very good sense. Patients are extremely appreciative when they can be treated quickly by a doctor they know and trust close to home.

Minor surgery for skin lesions is very satisfying: it gives you the opportunity to use the technical skills that are a part of being a doctor, it widens your scope as a GP, it increases your knowledge of dermatology, and of course it generates income for the practice. Provided you assess each patient individually and do not get out of your depth you are extremely unlikely to run into serious problems.

Managing skin lesions well is a rewarding, satisfying and enjoyable part of being a general practitioner.

Further reading

Brown, J. S. (1992) *Minor Surgery: A text and atlas*, 2nd edn, Chapman & Hall, London.

British Medical Association (1989) *A Code of Practice for Sterilization of Instruments and Control of Cross-infection*, British Medical Association, London.

Dando, P. (1993) *Medico-legal Aspects of Minor Surgery*, Medical Defence Union, London.

Champion, R. H., Burton, J. L. and Ebling, F. J. G. (eds) *Textbook of Dermatology*, 5th edn, Blackwell Scientific Publications, Oxford.

Index

Page numbers appearing in **bold** refer to figures, those appearing in ***bold italic*** refer to gallery entries and those appearing in *italic* refer to tables.